Women and Leadership
in Health Care

Catherine Robinson-Walker

Women and Leadership in Health Care

The Journey to Authenticity and Power

Jossey-Bass Publishers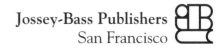
San Francisco

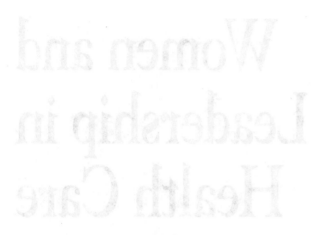

Jossey-Bass books and products are available through most bookstores. To contact Jossey-Bass directly, call (888) 378-2537, fax to (800) 605-2665, or visit our website at www.josseybass.com.

Substantial discounts on bulk quantities of Jossey-Bass books are available to corporations, professional associations, and other organizations. For details and discount information, contact the special sales department at Jossey-Bass.

 Manufactured in the United States of America on Lyons Falls Turin Book. This paper is acid-free and 100 percent totally chlorine-free.

Library of Congress Cataloging-in-Publication Data

Robinson-Walker, Catherine, 1946-
    Women and leadership in health care : the journey to
authenticity and power / Catherine Robinson-Walker. — 1st ed.
        p. cm.
    Includes bibliographical references and index.
    ISBN 0-7879-0933-5 (acid-free paper)
    1. Women in medicine.   2. Health care administrators.   3. Women
executives.   I. Title.
    R692 .R635 1999
    362.1'082—dc21

                                                                98-58078
                                                                CIP

FIRST EDITION
HB Printing   10 9 8 7 6 5 4 3 2

Contents

· ·

Preface

. . . .

Why do some women of undisputed talent opt out of the most senior roles in health care organizations? Why are some of them not even considered for these roles even if they are as qualified as men? And why do still others not seek the developmental opportunities that could prepare them for health care's top jobs?

These are just some of the compelling questions addressed in this book through dialogue with nearly one hundred women and men responsible for managing a significant portion of America's health care. As we enter the new millennium, we must confront an unavoidable reality: women are simply not present in the numbers we would expect, nor do they ascend at the rate we would expect to the most senior leadership roles in health care.

To understand this pernicious trend, we witness the sincere, forthcoming, and frank comments of this book's contributors as they offer their experiences, beliefs, and the context for their leadership practices. They air their convictions and concerns, describing gender's role in an industry that is filled with heart and commitment yet fraught with constantly conflicting demands on attention, resources, and priorities.

Every leader cited in this work is charged with powering an important aspect of the complex engine of health care. But here we learn that many are regularly suboptimized and frustrated in their ability to connect with and coordinate the resources in their charge.

Instead, they experience the ubiquitous reality of "fragmentation"—
the narrow confines, or *silos*, within which too much of health care
operates. Each devoutly singular department, discipline, and even
viewpoint unintentionally contributes to such fragmentation—
a serious phenomenon that may well be the single biggest barrier
to efficient, effective, and cost-conscious resource use in a public
concern that commands at least 15 percent of the Gross Domestic
Product of the United States.

How can any leader best address the true needs of those she
serves—individuals in search of health and care—when she experiences these barriers so frequently? Within this context we focus on
gender and its relevance to the leader's mandates. The contributors
to this book dig deeply into simple queries, posed in ways they could
have easily brushed aside. Instead, they chose to offer their views
with attention, consideration, and sincerity. We feel their trust, and
we are sobered and deeply informed by their telling observations.

As their witnesses, we are invited to listen generously and with
respect, whether their stories are "politically correct" or like our
own. Indeed, some or even many comments may not strike chords
with our own lives, nor with our beliefs about what others experience. But we are wise to remember that each contributor's vantage
point is unique, like ours. Taken together, their opinions crystallize,
guiding us to emerging patterns, new queries that deserve further
study, and answers to many concerns about gender's relevance to
leadership access and effectiveness in health care today. These rich
results also create new opportunities for further research with an
ever more diverse group of participants.

As the bearer of these truths, I hope that this book will benefit
each reader, as well as those who look to that reader for guidance and
those who will follow her in the years to come. I am not concerned
whether she is a prominent leader today. Rather, I hope that this
work inspires all readers about the role of leadership so that everyone, male or female, can assume the *stance of the leader* and the *call
to stewardship* no matter what her or his title.

The medium for most of this book is the story, for in story lies power—power to move us from our heads to our hearts, to places of feeling, action, and change. The stories in this work deserve our attention; they are told by accomplished professionals who together have created a wide and impressive swath of achievement in many health care arenas around the country. They operate on all rungs of the senior leadership ladder, extending their reach through vast organizational forms and purposes. Their venues range from community care settings to multibillion-dollar, multinational health care concerns.

Individually, they are well-trained physicians, nurses, public health experts, administrators, payers, consultants, executive recruiters, educators, and the like. Jointly, they render a rich portrait of the committed women and men who are at the helm of this huge and vital set of human services in the United States. They, along with key management experts, guide us to the skills, attitudes, and values that are most advantageous in traversing the scale of gender diversity from which the leader interacts every day.

When all is said and done, these voices lead us to a view of leadership beyond individual experiences, skills, and attitudes: leadership as being, leadership as character, and leadership as statement—simple, visionary, courageous, and profound. Here, we move past the questions and barriers of gender and away from a too-common view of health care management life today: beleaguered and handwringing. Instead, we see renewal, relearning, and working together as concepts that are not only voiced but lived. We join together as cocreators of a far better health care future formed as a natural, integrative outcome of collective wisdom born of difference and mutual respect. Here, we witness a far more compelling, transforming, and healthy vision for those in our care, and for ourselves.

This book presents a road map through and beyond concerns about gender, ending in a state where leadership flourishes through integrity and character, bolstered by the skills needed to get the job done. At its heart, this book is dedicated to balance, competence, and influence—all engaged in service of healing the health care system, the stewards of that system, and—most important—those in its care.

Book Overview

Part One of this work focuses on the key challenges of gender in health care. Chapter One considers the impact of gender on the efforts of male and female leaders and the paradox in our beliefs about gender's relationship to leadership. It introduces the 1997 Gender and Leadership in Healthcare Study—the vehicle for examining the compelling questions of gender's relevance. It also considers time and whether its mere passing is sufficient to close the gap between women's presence in management ranks and their presence in the highest posts.

Chapter Two considers the facts about women health care leaders; stumbling blocks women and men encounter as they move ahead; key values imbedded in the primary model of leadership in the 20th century in the United States; and new leadership paradigms and their relevance to gender. Chapter Three introduces the stories of the book's contributors: more than 90 percent of them believe gender plays a significant role in their own and others' leadership, and we learn in what ways this occurs. How do male and female expressions of stewardship differ, if they do, and how do these differences display themselves? And what happens when women and men don't conform to our expectations of their behaviors as leaders? Chapter Four helps us come to terms with the answers. We consider a host of gender-related dynamics and challenges and ways to address them that are followed up in Part Two.

Part Two highlights specific skills and behaviors that can help females in particular to excel in today's challenging and demanding environment. Chapter Five introduces gender's role in conflict, negotiation, and power. We review male and female approaches to disagreements and risk taking in health care encounters, ways to achieve common aims by promoting and managing difference, and new models of power along with ways to implement them.

Chapter Six focuses on communication, which for many leaders, inside and outside health care, is their most crucial skill. We review key socialization and communication differences between men and women on the job and focus on perceptions about some female leaders whose communication styles do not match those linked with clear and decisive leadership. We explore options and skills to mitigate these apparent mismatches in service of creating perceptions of competence, even when the dominant "male model" of leadership is at play.

Chapter Seven highlights career issues for female and male leaders, including the changing nature of work, jobs, and management; how women and men can maximize their own leadership opportunities in this environment; how women can manage the glass ceilings they still encounter; and how learning relates to leadership effectiveness in all these circumstances. Chapter Eight looks at renewal in both the personal and professional realms. We consider why we need it, why we don't do it, the costs of ignoring it, and the ways to bring it into our lives. It closes with a focus on mentoring—what it is, how it can be practiced successfully in health care, how it relates to gender, and how it can benefit us as mentors and as mentees.

Part Three puts it all together, moving us beyond challenges and barriers of gender—and even the specific skills that can counteract them—into a state of transformation and authenticity. Chapter Nine looks at the role gender plays as we evolve, examining several stages of mastery and wisdom individuals often pass through as they mature. It offers reflections on transformation and authenticity—what they are for the book's contributors and how significant they are to those who would fully mature as effective leaders. Chapter Ten brings us full circle, from the paradox of gender's impact in Chapter One to the power of moving through and beyond gender to leadership of consequence—no matter what our sex. We witness inspiring, heart-felt tales of stewardship born of integration and commitment summoned to stand up for what is right. We witness small and large acts of character and courage in the parting stories of the contributors.

The Audience

This work has been created for health care clinicians, executives, managers, healers, support personnel, and providers in all leadership roles, from clinical leadership to managers, supervisors, and care givers—all who are called upon to make decisions of import for and with the patients and resources on their watch. The book is crafted to speak to anyone who holds a coordinating role in administering care and health care services throughout this country. Academics, consultants, insurers, actuaries, staff in public health and policy agencies, foundation and association staff at the local, regional, state, and national levels—all may recognize the dimensions of their life's work in this discussion.

Those who are not yet in roles of responsibility will find value in these pages too. Very few twenty-somethings have yet landed in the positions of leadership that are the starting points for this probe. Still, their views were sought. Focus groups revealed that although students just five years ago were convinced that gender bias was a thing of the past, their postgraduate working experience has dramatically altered that belief.

Most importantly, this work is offered for both men and women. Many women are sure to find affinity with the female voices in the book, but men too will hear stories that bear witness to their own lives and callings.

Let us begin.

Acknowledgments

I am filled with gratitude and respect for the countless souls who have helped me create this work. For her unwavering and uplifting support during the four plus years of this project, I shall always be in Rebecca McGovern's debt. First my editor at Jossey-Bass, then my independent developmental editor, Becky shared my vision for this book, making each step ahead appear possible, if not downright easy. Special thanks too for her careful choice of meeting spots— gathering in bookstores over the months, then years, offered me continuing proof that books do indeed come into being.

To everyone who participated in the 1997 Gender and Leadership in Healthcare Study, I am eternally grateful. Without exception, each granted me a trusted glimpse of the sincere beliefs, history, and hopes we share for a new future. Without each woman and man who participated, the book would be missing fibers from its texture and pieces of our emerging understanding of the relationship between gender and leadership in health care today.

Who would have thought a writer could actually love the work of an editor? My editor in charge of cutting with vision and discernment was Christina Van Horn. Her competence, her perennially cheerful songs by email on all those mornings at dawn, and her constant belief in this work earn her my greatest appreciation.

Thanks, too, to the team at Jossey-Bass for their expertise, to my research assistant Stephanie Fish, and to the many health care stewards with whom I have been privileged to work in these past twenty-five years. In them, I have found mentors, role models, and a plethora of examples of commitment to leadership at its best.

Finally, my heartfelt thanks to my husband, Tim, and my family and friends for their abiding faith and patience. Who knew the muse could be so enduring?

The Author

· ·

Catherine Robinson-Walker is executive director of The Academy for Healthcare Quality, a collaborative venture of the Joint Commission on Accreditation of Healthcare Organizations and five leading universities throughout the United States. She is a pioneer in conceiving breakthrough strategies for leadership and executive education in health care. As founding executive director of the Network for Healthcare Management, Robinson-Walker partnered for two decades with national and international health care executives, associations, and distinguished universities to create innovative leadership resources.

Her widely recognized successes range from collaborating to create the first computer-based master's degree program for health management in the mid-1980s to the first Center for Health Management Research sponsored by the National Science Foundation, fifteen major universities, and a dozen of the largest health systems in the United States.

Robinson-Walker has also served as a leadership program consultant to national organizations such as the VHA, Inc., a 1400-hospital consortium; the American Organization for Nurse Executives (AONE); and the Hill-Rom Corporation. Working with AONE, Hill-Rom, and nurse leaders throughout the country, she co-created the national Center for Nursing Leadership in the late 1990s.

Robinson-Walker holds a bachelor's degree in psychology and sociology from DePauw University in Greencastle, Indiana. While earning her master's degree in business administration in the Executive Program at Golden Gate University in San Francisco, she was awarded the Warren A. Pillsbury Honors Scholarship for academic achievement. She has received many honors throughout her career, ranging from invitations to serve as a Founding Board Member of Leadership California to sponsored participation in Leadership America, and Women, Leadership and the Future. Most recently, Robinson-Walker was selected as "1998 Woman of the Year" by Women Healthcare Executives of Northern California/The American College of Healthcare Executives.

She is a frequent speaker on trends and strategies for stewardship in health care, and the path to power and effectiveness for women.

Women and Leadership
in Health Care

To my teachers, in their many forms

Part I

· ·

Coming to Terms with Gender

1

. . . .

The Paradox of Gender

Is effective leadership in health care based on or determined by gender? No, say prolific authors who have long studied leadership, my own mentors through more than twenty years of executive development practice, and scores of leaders I interviewed for the study on which this book is based.

But when does no mean yes? When the executives interviewed for this work were asked whether they believe gender plays a major role in health care leadership in general, and in their own leadership practices in particular, nearly all said yes!

This chapter examines this paradox, which leapt from the interviews of the 1997 Gender and Leadership in Healthcare Study (GLHS) that I developed to investigate gender's relevance to health care leadership. Underscoring the importance of this paradox is the continuing dearth of females in the most senior posts, despite a political and social climate that paves the way for their presence.

Exact numbers change rapidly, of course, but as of 1999 women simply are not present in senior management positions to the extent that we would expect when 85 percent of U.S. health care workers are female. This disparity is found not only in this field but also in senior management strata throughout the United States, regardless of field. As of 1996, women filled nearly a third of all management roles, but the majority are positions with relatively little power and authority (Klenke, 1996, p. 17).

Nearly one hundred leading male and female health care executives of various disciplines, including medicine, nursing, and management, participated in the GLHS. In the main, their ages range from forty-one to fifty-five—what one would expect for individuals in senior leadership roles. Their organizations and communities of practice include national and regional health systems; integrated delivery organizations; academic institutions; national associations representing management and clinical professions; public health concerns; executive recruiting companies; foundation staff; worldwide consulting firms; and suppliers of health care products. (For a partial list of study participants, see Appendix A.)

The broad demographics of senior female leaders throughout the health care sector reflect, disturbingly, far fewer women than we could expect given their prominence throughout the system and their importance as buyers and recipients of care. These data, coupled with the study participants' perceptions, set up a compelling paradox: we say health care leadership is not gender based, but women in significant numbers do not occupy positions of leadership, power, and authority.

The possible reasons for this paradox are disquieting, and they would be even more so if there were no viable ways for women (and men) to move through and beyond it. I wrote this book as a map for navigating gender challenges based on the well-considered recommendations, tried and true practices, and numerous tips for success from the study contributors and leading authors. This chapter discusses:

- Gender's relationship to diversity

- The impact of gender on the efforts of prominent male and female health care leaders

- Examination of the "pipeline" theory of women's advancement

- Initial exploration of beliefs about gender's importance

- Study contributors' hypotheses about whether gender's significance is changing with the times

To begin, *gender* can be defined in many ways. For this work we shall use this rich interpretation: "Gender is a social construct built of traditions, language and symbols that can create deep affiliation and deep division among people. We chant about the benefits of diversity, yet sometimes we stumble among the traditions, language and symbols that can create deep divides among even this most basic of sub-cultures: male and female ways of leading, communicating and getting the work of healthcare accomplished" (Klenke, 1996, p. 15).

Gender is but one aspect of the ubiquitous issue of diversity. It coexists with race, social class, ethnicity, family of origin, profession, and education, to name just a few of an individual's defining characteristics. Each one forms uniquely in every human being and adds to the complexity of the health care steward's task. She must provide effective leadership for her disparate peers and colleagues, her staff and team members, her department, her organization, her community, or her health care system. At the same time, she must thrive as a leader even as perceptions about gender may contribute to projections and misperceptions regarding her own and others' intent and competence.

Notable in the GLHS, many contributors reported a significant level of gender-related "discord" that they believe has an impact on a leader's effectiveness. Acclaimed management scholar Judith Rosener's term for this discord is "sexual static." Rosener (1995) likens sexual static to TV or radio interference, causing impediments for the messages being communicated. She concludes that such noise creates discomfort for men and frustration for women. It is so important, says Rosener, that men unconsciously exclude women from the executive suite because of this discomfort.

Several female GLHS participants are convinced that the noise and the effect of gender within their exercise of leadership in health care is "always present, in every interaction." Interestingly, no men made this statement.

One GLHS contributor observes from her vantage point of thirty years in a successful national consulting practice: "I have seen male business leaders become male board members who hire male executives, resulting in male-dominated purchasers and payers who see nothing odd about male-dominated organizations. Often they are insensitive to the ways in which the healthcare system is hostile and uncaring toward women."

There are powerful incubators in which the conscious and unconscious cultural biases of men and women grow and flourish. For example, the tradition, training, standards, and values of the medical, nursing, and allied health professions, which have well served health care consumers, have also produced cultures that can unwittingly be closed to those other than "their own." This inadvertent but narrow world view can limit the success of multimembership teams that must work interdependently for the well-being of patients, consumers, organizations, and themselves.

For example, a seasoned female physician, well-regarded leader, and GLHS contributor believes that the physician culture is highly territorial and a hybrid of corporate and medical culture: "Medical culture is very male dominated. . . . [W]hen you marry that with corporate culture (e.g. male dominated and hierarchical), this is dominance 'squared.' As a female, you must be more compliant and cooperative to get anywhere."

Nurses, too, observe the omnipresent effect of gender within their culture. The words of one GLHS interviewee represent many: "It is simply impossible for nurses to not pay attention to gender. It is the classic nurse/physician issue. In the last twenty years, there are more female doctors, and higher level nurses. Yet, the dynamic 'I'm your boss. I am the decision maker' is always there."

Is Time the Elixir?

Do women and men need to concern themselves with the continuing facts of women's absence at the highest levels of leadership in health care? Or will the trend reverse itself? The often-heard current rationale for the dearth of women at the top of the health care workforce is the "pipeline theory." Many women and men believe that with enough time, women will be represented in accordance with their numbers. As they season and gather experience, they will assume key roles in the totals we would expect, in the time we would expect, and in proportion to their abilities.

But the 1995 American College of Healthcare Executives (ACHE) study (detailed in Chapter Two), which compared the career attainments of male and female health care executives, suggests this may not be true. This study reports that "as they age, women health care executives continued to experience lower career attainments compared to men and, in fact, the gap between the two gender groups has grown over the past five years" (American College of Healthcare Executives, 1996, p. 4).

Indeed, the gap gets bigger as women age. Dr. Cynthia Carter Haddock, coauthor of the ACHE study, asks a critical question: "How long do women have to wait—30, 40, 50 years? No one's career is that long! By the late 1970s and early 1980s women were significant in numbers in graduate programs [in health administration]. Yet, as of today . . . they have not attained the levels of leadership that their male counterparts have."

The Gender and Leadership in Healthcare Study

Against the backdrop of this important evidence, the GLHS posed a series of related questions. The first was straightforward: Does gender play a major role in health care leadership? Ninety-two percent of the study's respondents believe gender does play a major role in health care leadership. Four individuals, or 5 percent, do not believe this is the case, and several (3 percent) said they did not know. Males and females responded nearly identically.

Rich comments about this nearly uniform belief of gender's importance provide key insights. First, people answered this question quite differently in tone and degree of certainty. For many, the answer was a resounding "absolutely." Those who were less than certain cited other factors such as context. Several others "are beginning to" believe gender exerts a considerable measure of importance in executive practice.

Leland R. Kaiser, Ph.D., is a noted futurist who has consulted with hundreds of health care organizations nationally over the last twenty years. As a GLHS contributor, his view of the health care system in this regard is uncompromising: "I have never witnessed a healthcare organization that was gender-indifferent. The degree to which gender plays a role in leadership practice in modern healthcare varies with the organization."

To be sure, many females do play highly significant roles in medicine, nursing, the allied health professions, community health, management, and policy, to name just a few. But at the senior leadership level, the story is often different.

Eunice Azzani, a partner in the prominent executive recruiting firm Korn/Ferry International, San Francisco, is a specialist in not-for-profit leadership placement. She minces no words: "The ceiling for women healthcare leaders is a hard plastic one." Azzani confirms the evidence: the discussion is about the composition of the ceiling for women—not whether it exists.

The research experience of GLHS contributor Lawton R. Burns, a professor at the Wharton School at the University of Pennsylvania, supports this: "Between 1994 and 1996, a colleague and I conducted a study of major full-service, integrated health care systems in the United States, particularly in the West and Midwest. We asked to speak to the systems' senior leaders, yet we interviewed very few women."

A highly influential male consultant sums up the situation bluntly: "Clearly women do not play a major role in management in this field." Convinced that this is an artifact of the sociological legacy of medicine, he believes that "health care organizations have become the 'utilities' of medical practice. Women are in supporting positions for those practices. Nursing, for example, is a ghetto, in sociological terms."

This lack of significant female presence in senior leadership roles was not always the case. Sister Mary Jean Ryan, president and CEO of SSM Health System headquartered in St. Louis, Missouri, reminds us that the first health care leaders early in the 20th century were women—nuns, nurses, and others. Then, in the early 1920s, an emphasis on a business mentality emerged and men were placed in these positions. "Nuns were considered to be sweet little things, who couldn't run a healthcare facility," she says.

The Context and Challenge for Health Care Organizations

Why aren't women accelerating to leadership prominence, despite good intentions, the passage of time, beliefs to the contrary, and a compelling political climate? What follows are brief suggestions, which Chapters Two and Four will augment.

The Survival Imperative

The news media today are replete with a never-ending flow of public concern about health care, spurred particularly by the advent of managed care. Although this apprehension is more than justified, such public attention adds to the already significant pressures faced by physicians, nurses, executives, and other health care workers. Every day, they are implored to do more with less, satisfy increasingly diverse populations with expanding demands for service and quality, and stretch insufficient resources among numerous deserving, yet competing, groups.

Those I interviewed raised this dynamic frequently—often in the context of beliefs that certain leadership roles are disappearing in this world of less funding and more service demands. For at least six GLHS contributors, such realities contribute to an atmosphere of less risk taking and greater need for organizational survival. They believe such factors seriously impair even the best efforts to recruit and place talented women in high-level positions.

A GLHS contributor who is a public health leader in the east offered a distressing example. Late for our interview, he apologized by saying, "I just received word from the Mayor's office that two-thirds of my staff will be cut. The Mayor also declared that it is public health week, in part because of the excellent job the Department is doing!"

The Importance of Place

As noted in the Preface, every setting in which health care leadership is exercised is unique, and not all settings are equal. For example, GLHS contributor Donna Fosbinder conducted a survey of nurse executives in 1995 in the southwest. She succinctly describes the results: "The glass ceiling is stopping nurses at every level." The same can hold true in a midwest corporate setting. Another GLHS contributor notes, "I moved from the Chief Nursing Officer position of an 850-bed hospital—a powerful position—to a corporate position. This was considered a step 'forward,' yet this position was not a strategic position at the corporate level. Rather, I functioned as staff, preparing for accreditation visits and the like."

Lest we believe that the challenge of obtaining leadership roles does not exist for female physicians, another contributor, a prominent female physician operating at a national health policy level, refers not to a "glass ceiling" for female doctors, but to a "lexan" ceiling. Translation: this is a bulletproof model!

Some health care settings appear to have less history to overcome and are better able to open their doors to women. Robert Boyle, a past chairman of the Medical Group Management Association (MGMA), observes striking differences between hospitals and ambulatory care clinics. "Hospitals are more traditional and hierar-chical—roles have more stereotypical definitions. In clinics, how-ever, nursing has strong roles, and clinicians work arm-in-arm. Women are managing, and there are more nurse-doctor teams."

Women also hold more leadership positions in managed-care organizations and in physician practices. However, Boyle points out, this changes as the physician group increases in size: "At around 25 to 50 physicians, groups usually have male leadership, and women have secondary roles." At the national level, he sees MGMA's female leaders generally emerging from smaller group practices.

Community settings make a difference as well. For example, one male senior executive of a large for-profit national health organiza-tion observes that females are better represented at higher levels of these institutions than they are at the community level.

The Ubiquitous Double Standard

Management theorist Judith Rosener believes that all women lead-ers face a difficult challenge: when behaviors associated with females are considered negative or valueless, gender is seen as relevant. Yet when other behaviors associated with women are considered val-uable or positive, gender is not seen as relevant (Rosener, 1995, p. 12). (See Chapter Two for in-depth discussion.)

GLHS interviewees offered many examples of this double stan-dard for women in health care leadership. Fred Graham, a senior executive with MGMA for twenty years, provided perspective on his experience: "If women do display the same 'successful' charac-teristics as the male, they are not welcomed, or sought for the senior management team. If they are competent, yet have excellent peo-ple skills, they are treated differently—they are given less 'rope.'"

A woman who founded her company many years ago finds that even in her successful consulting practice, gender is a continuing subtext: "I am aware that my Board, even though I am the co-founder of my organization and quite experienced, looks on me as a woman in need of direction, and 'uppity' if I contradict anything members say, even when it is erroneous."

At least a half-dozen GLHS interviewees mentioned another twist to this aspect of the gender paradox. Myra Isenhart, who focuses on communication and conflict within health care and other businesses, hears an important complaint frequently from female physicians: "In meetings, a woman will come up with an idea, and it's a man who gets the credit when he mentions it later in the meeting." A female CEO of a major system reiterates this, adding, "Does this speak to women learning to operate effectively with regard to communications and stature differences? It probably does." (Chapter Five describes this phenomenon in sociological terms; Chapter Six discusses options for moving through communication challenges such as this.)

The Unconvinced

About 8 percent of the GLHS respondents did not agree that gender plays a major role in leadership in health care. Their views offer insight into the complexity of the question and the importance of the leader's vantage point when answering it.

"Gender is overblown," states one contributor. "All we care about is output." Another GLHS contributor, a female in a role of facilitating direct care in her community, believes that gender isn't the issue. "Certain topics [such as gender] can detract from leadership accountability." she says. "For some it's an excuse to play a role."

One male clearly stated that it's not one sex or the other that is the focus for health care leaders: "Capabilities are the issue—core capabilities and competencies are the issue." He offers us a glimpse of the paradox. Few would argue his point. But if this is the case, why aren't women in significant numbers in positions of significant leadership responsibility?

Clearly a barrier does exist. A physician and leading educator with substantial health policy experience suggests that we do not know the answer to the question "Does gender play a major role?"

In his own educational institution there are "good numbers of women students," but "you don't see them coming through to top leadership levels. It's more than just 'needing more time.' There's a barrier to feminization at the top."

Gender's Significance Today

Is gender's relevance to women's access to and success in senior leadership positions shifting? When asked whether and how gender's influence is changing, GLHS contributors hold beliefs that can be aggregated in the following ways.

Women's Future Is Increasingly Bright

This future is solidly rooted in the well-acknowledged acceptance of females as the caregivers of choice for many consumers of health care. In *An Unfinished Revolution* (Friedman, 1994), noted economist Eli Ginzberg observes that female doctors spend more time talking with their patients. This has been shown to increase patient satisfaction, and Ginzberg and others believe it will ultimately lower medical costs as well.

A longtime recruiter in the San Francisco Bay area sees increasing demand for female family practice physicians. Why? In part because "females want females," and females are often the purchasers of health care for their families. A practicing female physician in the Rocky Mountains says there is a huge demand for her services, as well as those of the other female doctors in her organization.

Patrick G. Hays, president and CEO of the national Blue Cross/Blue Shield Association, believes gender's significance is greater now because of the dawning awareness regarding women and children and their centrality to health care. "It is difficult to 'walk the walk' unless you've been there. . . . [T]here can be a disconnect with the 50 year old white male."

Several other GLHS contributors noticed similar effects of gender on medicine. Lillee Gilenas is the senior nurse executive at the system level of VHA, Inc., a 1,400-hospital consortium: "With more women in physician roles, there is a greater prominence of issues such as family life and children. Women are making their presence known. This is not the norm, but I do observe [their presence] as pushing the envelope in training and in practice." Diane Littlefield, director of the Women's Health Leadership Program in Sacramento, California, also sees the value for health system leadership as women enter who are motivated by the goals of family and community health. "Female decision making tends to be more inclusive and, as a result, policies are more appropriate for communities, and for women and family services."

GLHS contributor Molly Joel Coye, former health commissioner in New Jersey and director of the California Health Department, perceives these strengths, too: "As nurturers, women have an advantage in understanding both service and market needs. As we move to consumer-driven care, away from doctor- and provider-driven care, women leaders also have the advantage because they *are* the market—they comprise 60–70 percent of the decision makers for the family's health."

Hays adds a profoundly important observation: "Managed care has become derailed from its original intent—there is a need and opportunity for women, who have a different approach, but get the same result."

GLHS contributor Wanda Jones is a nationally respected futurist and population-based planning expert. She and other experts see the growing independence of females in numerous health care settings. From self-governance models that many nursing departments have adapted to the growth of home care and case management, nurses have gained in the scopes of their practice while offering their significant skills in patient-focused care and case management. Women also dominate some pre- and post-acute health agencies, such as Planned Parenthood, which is run largely by women.

Where there is still a shortage of some types of physicians, the demand for organized primary care has exploded, thus producing opportunities for nurse practitioners and extended-practice nurses. Alternative therapies, the growing use of complementary healing and wellness practices, and care offered in nontraditional settings also offer women new opportunities for significant leadership roles.

Some Women Are Stepping Around the Barriers

Joseph M. Hafey, executive director of the Public Health Institute, a multimillion-dollar national venture offering infrastructure for public health initiatives across the country, sees the leadership potential for women becoming reality, at least in some spheres. For women, he says, "There are very few opportunities to enter a lot of traditional places of work—e.g., large corporations and universities" but it "is pretty easy to appoint yourself director of an emerging organization. When women look creatively at employment in health care now, this opens more leadership opportunities for them."

Elaina Genser, M.P.H., an executive search consultant since 1984, remembers a time not long ago when recruiters would ask their clients if women would be acceptable. But now, she says, "People are trying consciously to balance their teams, not only in gender, but with clinical and non-clinical personnel."

Carol Spain Woltring, a keen observer of both national and international public health leadership, adds: "The changes that are occurring are creating opportunities, new roles, redefining businesses. There is more need to work in communities." Women will find very good opportunities there, she points out, especially if they are patient with the process of asking community members to define the problem rather than telling them what it is.

Now the head of his own consulting firm, a male contributor who was also a successful chief operating officer within a large not-for-profit health system in California says there are more women in executive positions now. "At a large competitor, where the health care world is like Bosnia, the executive head is a female," he points out. "People are looking for people with strong capabilities."

For Others, Barriers Are Still in Place

Still, a number of GLHS contributors felt less optimistic that gender's significance was waning. A female public health official states, "While gender plays a more positive role than it did 20 years ago, this doesn't negate its importance now." Leland Kaiser concurs, adding, "It is still present and will be for many years. But, we have made a lot of progress, attributable largely to the passage of sexual harassment legislation and the increasing frequency of gender discrimination suits."

One GLHS contributor, an executive recruiter, states: "There are a few places where they really want female candidates, but they are having trouble finding qualified people." She then touches on two issues we will discuss further in Chapter Two: that women often don't want leadership positions, and that "boards want a 'person like us.'"

For Some, Barriers Are Even Greater

There are also those who believe that gender barriers are more significant now than in the immediate past. Some interviewees believe this is a response to consolidation and the need to do more with less amidst calls for greater accountability. Other reasons cited include the following:

The Unionization of Professions

Lawton R. Burns notes, "Unionization of these professions, such as nursing, and even medicine, is in response to the heavy-handed corporate control as mergers in health care progress." Some in professional positions pursue this course because they perceive such consolidation as compromising their ability to deliver high quality care to their patients.

For Some, It's Survival

The chief nurse of a major national health care entity cites the concern many executives share: "There are now more survival games in place. Although we mouth one thing, regarding gender, I do not see that much difference." A male public health expert agrees: "I sense the hospital/HMO environment now is 'all or nothing, survival of the fittest, give me the silver bullet.' Perhaps in five years, there will be an atmosphere in which really good people will be given the chances." Public health care is different, he adds, because it "has not seen the massive restructuring that acute health care is experiencing."

Isolation of Health Care

A number of contributors observe that health care hasn't been that competitive in the last twenty to thirty years. Molly Joel Coye, M.D., is among them: "There has been a subtle dismissal of health care in business schools, because it has been atypical of the rest of the economy, with cost-based reimbursement and the very different marketing for hospitals versus consumer products." Contributor Eunice Azzani adds, "There is a certain elitism [in health care], not unlike high tech. Health care traditionally has not been willing to look at individual [candidates] from outside. Merely recycling the same people just recycles the problems too. Maybe if we'd been able to bring new people into the field, we could have avoided the 'crash and burn' state health care is in now."

Six of One, Half a Dozen of Another

Several contributors perceive that gender today is neither more significant nor less. One female commented that, in her medium-sized city, "I look around, and I see the same people running health care organizations. There is only one woman."

For others, it is health care's culture that has not changed. Says one female interviewee: "Men are more into power, particularly with mergers and acquisitions. But patient care suffers." Another contributor believes a glass ceiling still exists at the top "because of the male inclination to dominate. In my experience with boards of directors, many men know there are more competent women than the men who are on them."

Summing Up

This chapter introduces the gender paradox in health care leadership, the myths and convictions we hold about that paradox, and our beliefs about its salience in the future. We can conclude that although the future for women leaders is hopeful, progress in attaining top leadership posts is slow. There is little doubt that the future for women in care giving roles is secure, and the groundwork for attaining positions of significant leadership responsibility is laid. Yet there are still real concerns about when women will arrive in these positions.

The next chapter provides greater consideration of the leadership models and values that often prevail in health care, and offers a glimpse of the barriers that can result when women bring different approaches to their work.

Gender, Values, and Leadership

Chapter One explored perceptions and beliefs about whether and how gender has an impact on health care leadership practice. Chapter Two offers the reader context for these beliefs by investigating the following:

1. The facts about women leaders in health care interpreted from the 1995 ACHE gender and careers study

2. Stumbling blocks women face regarding access to key leadership roles

3. Values that have been inbred in the primary model of leadership for most of the 20th century

4. Application of those values in health care settings

5. Emerging leadership paradigms and how they may take hold as the transformation of health care proceeds

Examining the Data

The American College of Healthcare Executives (ACHE) conducted significant research projects in 1990 and 1995 to shed light on gender and careers as experienced within its thirty thousand members. Particularly instructive for this inquiry are the results of the 1995 study *A Comparison of the Career Attainments of Men and*

Women Healthcare Executives. According to Weil and others (1996), the conclusions were the following:

1. Women still earned less than men. Nearly half the 386 women surveyed reported that sometime in the last five years they were denied fair compensation because of their gender; none of the 323 men reported similar discrimination. Also, although women had attained equal levels of education and experience, they earned an average of $15,000, or about 16 percent, less than their male counterparts. This was a slight improvement over 1990.

2. Women and men experienced similar job satisfaction.

3. Women were as likely as men to be promoted within their organizations, but only 8 percent of the women in the study, compared with 21 percent of the men, were CEOs.

4. Stereotypes of male or female leadership attributes still lingered. Fifty-three percent of men and 82 percent of women perceived women as demonstrating more nurturing skills, whereas both groups saw men as competitive, assertive risk takers who benefit more from advancement opportunities. Yet 57 percent of men and 69 percent of women believed that men and women are equal in their leadership qualities.

5. Twenty-nine percent of women and 5 percent of men said they had been sexually harassed in the workplace in the last five years. These figures match those of other industries. Also, as were employees in many industries, men and women are concerned with job security and the futures of their careers.

6. Women reported more home and family obligations than men did. As previous studies of managerial women have found, women were more likely to be the primary caregivers and more often yielded their career advancement to opportunities offered to their spouses. Yet career interruptions of three or

more months did not markedly diminish women's salaries in comparison to salaries of women without interrupted careers.

7. The gender gap may be narrowing in some areas. ACHE stated that there were evident improvements noted when comparing the 1995 data with the data of the 1990 study. Thirty-eight percent of women in the 1995 study reported being the first females to occupy their current positions. They were also more satisfied with the support they receive from their bosses and the promotion opportunities available to them.

8. Women reported in 1995 that they were less satisfied with the support they receive from their male colleagues than are their counterparts. Men simply "don't see" that they are given preferential treatment; given this difference in perception, women can conclude that there is a lack of support from their male colleagues.

Stumbling Blocks for Women at the Top

Females in the 1995 ACHE study believe "something is there" with respect to gender barriers. For example, to the statement "I feel discriminated against in obtaining a better position because of my gender," 30 percent of the females responded in the affirmative, as contrasted to 4 percent of the men. How much changed since ACHE's 1990 study? Then, 35 percent of women and 2 percent of men agreed with the statement.

Interviews from the 1997 GLHS provide insight into why women may not have access to, or choose to pursue, positions at the highest levels of leadership. In considering these possibilities, we are advised to appreciate the complexity of gender and the difficulty of distinguishing its discrete role in inquiries about the components of effective health care leadership. Janet Bickel, vice president of the Association of American Medical Colleges, for example, describes confounding factors that can hinder one's career progress as "accumulating advantages and disadvantages." She notes that, as in other fields, many variables contribute to one's career development and success in health care. The results of any leader's efforts are never the sum of just one factor. Rather, they are products of many influences that accumulate in force over time (Friedman, 1994, p. 228).

Gender, then, and the other variables that are briefly considered may not be the sole contributing factors to females' realization of leadership aims. With that understanding, we can consider possible difficulties women may face in attaining senior positions.

Stumbling Block One: Assumption that Time is the Answer

Chapter One focused on the common belief that is well articulated by a male GLHS contributor: "Many of us assume that the women are . . . in the pipelines—in medical school, health administration programs, and other preparatory fields such as business and law. Soon, they will be in the lower and later in the senior management and leadership positions simply by virtue of their presence." As we saw in Chapter One, however, time alone may not be sufficient to assure the presence of women in senior roles.

Stumbling Block Two: Do Women Want the Top Jobs?

As women's careers progress, they tend to advance more slowly than men with similar experience and education. In the 1995 ACHE study, for example, well over twice as many men as women had attained CEO positions, although women and men were just as likely to be promoted within their organizations. The study reported that half as many women said they aspire to CEO positions.

For the GLHS, Cynthia Carter Haddock, coauthor of the 1995 ACHE study, comments on the question of women's desire for CEO and other senior-most positions: "These findings could indicate that there really are barriers to women achieving the most senior positions in healthcare organizations. Perhaps women do not choose to pursue these positions. If that is the case, is it because they perceive the barriers to these positions, and/or because they have other priorities in their lives?"

GLHS contributor Patrick Hays, president and CEO of Blue Cross and Blue Shield nationwide, offered his perspective based on his longtime experience as president and CEO of Sutter Health. In the latter part of the 1980s, Sutter, a highly successful integrated health system in California, fostered a very strong work culture and high expectations, says Hays. Fast-track women executives were saying that they didn't want to go higher in the organization because of the demands that Sutter placed on them. Committed to understanding the issue, Hays commissioned a study on the corporate culture, which uncovered a number of forceful comments that answered his question.

To the question "Why don't you want to move up, even though Hays and his lieutenants think you're a star?" the women said that senior management culture at Sutter was "Give all, do whatever it takes—success is everything." Hays notes, "It was interesting—for males, chests puffed up—implying 'a fine organization, of course, we're a fine organization.' What was a source of pride for white males was a major disabler for others."

Stumbling Block Three: What Is Appropriate Behavior to Attain Senior Leadership Roles?

Haddock concludes that whereas men will say they want to be CEO, women may keep their ambitions to themselves because they don't feel it is appropriate to do otherwise. "Based on the current data," she says, "It is possible to conclude that there are real barriers to women becoming CEOs, and that implicitly or explicitly women understand this. This may have an impact on their performance and their careers."

Stumbling Block Four:
Are Female Candidates Considered Fairly?

One female GLHS contributor has worked with hundreds of hospital trustees, and she observes palpable board retrenchment in recent years. "They are moving back to male-dominated Boards, and the new nominees are frequently all men," she says. "At the same time, the skill set many boards are seeking is business-oriented," the default assumption of many being that men have the required skills. Several male contributors said the same thing, one putting it most bluntly: "I sit on a number of boards, and when we are hiring, it becomes clear that no females need apply."

Stumbling Block Five: Who Points the Way?

Are women being counseled to seek the most prominent leadership positions and fields of endeavor within health care? It is common knowledge that many career counselors in medical schools direct women into primary care, traditionally the lower-paying and lower-status profession for physicians. Rosener (1995) and others suggest that by doing this we deepen our already burgeoning two-tier medical care system of male specialists and female primary caregivers.

A number of women who are forty and older commented that early on they perceived their career choices to be severely limited by gender. GLHS contributor Pam Bromley's comments reflect those of others: "I felt I had only three career choices: teaching, clerical and nursing." Her parents agreed, even refusing to pay her way through school if she did not stick with nursing.

Stumbling Block Six: Parenting

One GLHS senior male executive says it all for many women and some men: "This issue compromises many career choices"—a trend he sees as likely to continue. Nationally recognized economist Victor R. Fuchs of Stanford University agrees: "The economic disparity between men and woman stems from the conflict between

work and family rather than from career investment patterns. . . .
The cost to women of combining work and family is a cost not
borne equally by men" (Rosener, 1995, p. 62).

GLHS contributor Carla Wiggins, whose 1994 University of
Minnesota doctoral dissertation focused on career attainment among
male and female health care managers, says what many other contributors also voiced: "Women try hard to keep it all separate—the
50–60 hours of work and everything else." But reality requires a new
approach, she adds: "We should be integrating the elements in our
lives, rather than separating them." (Chapter Seven looks more
closely at ideas and perspectives for balancing careers and families.)

Stumbling Block Seven:
Do Women Have Role Models and Mentors?

Some GLHS interviewees speculate that females who do not reach
senior leadership positions lack role models and mentors, although
a number of the successful women in the GLHS did have female
role models at some point in their early personal or professional
lives. For example, one highly successful female nurse executive
noted that in her large extended family, thirty nurses, men and
women, served as her role models and mentors.

The importance of models and mentors should not be down-
played. Their absence may significantly contribute to women's near
absence at the top in health care. As one GLHS contributor says,
"Women are not mentored, and without it, they find it so difficult
to progress that they give up the trip."

Stumbling Block Eight: Taking on "Male" Characteristics

Heidi Boerstler, who directs the University of Colorado's graduate
programs in health administration, says, "Women make a big mistake when they copy male behaviors. For example, people respond
to men who run autocratic meetings—it's okay, but men are uncomfortable with women acting like men." But a female physician comments that women who have "come up through the ranks" were

coached by men. She considers this an advantage because "They can take on the attributes considered to be more [masculine], yet at the same time tap into their own attributes, including being more inclusive, and exhibiting vulnerability."

But a dearth of female role models and mentors can easily create an imbalance in the behaviors and qualities women witness and incorporate into their own leadership portfolios. One prominent female who has served on several boards of directors points out that women physicians she's observed reacting negatively to the environment are not willing to "do time" in state and national political structures. They not only do not elect to serve as leaders, but they also do not serve as models for younger colleagues.

It is also important to recognize the important contribution men have made to many females as they have advanced. Consider, for example, Patricia Cahill, president and CEO of Catholic Health Initiatives, a multibillion-dollar health system in the Rocky Mountains and western United States. She has benefited from a career-long pattern of support from men that has been important to her success. Through these relationships, Pat has come to understand the need to "cast your own shadow."

Stumbling Block Nine: Once Promoted, Then What?

Some women do make that step into higher management echelons, but what work do they do? One male leader of a multinational health concern is joined by others in observing that women are often the chief operating officers, the less "glamorous" or "glory" positions. "It has been a long time since true operations was the supply chain [for senior leadership positions]," he says.

Well-regarded GLHS contributor Roxane Spitzer is an accomplished health care executive and prolific author. She agrees that many women still carry the day-to-day responsibilities, and confirms that women are more apt to be in marketing, volunteer departments, nursing, public relations, human resources, and community outreach than in finance, medical staff development, fund-raising, or board leadership.

Today's Health Care Environment

To understand the interplay of gender, leadership, and health care, we must move them into the bigger picture. As we saw in Chapter One, the ways medical care is delivered and even the definition of care itself are radically transforming, economically and systemically. This is occurring within the complicated contradictions of growing community needs, tighter funding, and conflicting consumer, organizational, and payor demands. At the same time, the expectations of Americans of high-quality, affordable, and accessible health care have never been greater. At times these important but confounding economic, social, and ethical imperatives may seem irreconcilable. Health care's leaders become susceptible to confusion, exhaustion, disenchantment, and ever-increasing demands on their time. At the same time, their learning needs and their professional and personal expectations for excellence and reward for a job well done are often compromised. Too often, it is against this backdrop that the leader's responsibilities are rendered.

The Limitations of Gender Typing

Much controversy exists about sex differences in behaviors, attitudes, and styles, whether they are biologically or culturally determined—or both—and whether and how they differ between men and women.

We may gain wisdom by reflecting on the "shorthand" that is frequently used to categorize individuals and their actions. *Stereotypes* are generalizations that we use to describe groups, characteristics, and behaviors. Stereotypes are frequently strong, influential, unconscious, and crippling. They often lead to, or are based on, oversimplifications about particular groups and the people within them.

Stereotypical qualities of women, for example, include likability, affection, soft-spokenness, selflessness, giving, yielding easily, compassion, listening, fairness, and process orientation. Common political stereotypes are less favorable: if a female leads in a commanding way, she can be considered overly aggressive, obnoxious, overbearing. But if women conform to the stereotypical female behaviors of passivity, nurturance, and cooperation, they are viewed as weak, submissive, and unable to lead successfully. To men we attribute competitiveness, decisiveness, action orientation, aggression, self-reliance, strength, independence, ambition, and dominance.

Taken as dichotomies and in the extreme, these stereotypical qualities paint an antiquated picture of female and male domains: home and hearth, nurturing and giving for women; public life, sports and military, or competition and domination for men. Creating new, more politically acceptable stereotypes for men and women merely displaces the old with the modern rather than promoting freedom and a continuum of skills and behaviors for both men and women. Worse, these stereotypes don't call forth the possibilities held in the breadth of differences between and within male and female leaders.

Stereotypes have other important limitations. For example, as we obtain new information about people other than their sex, we begin to discriminate at levels beyond gender. To illustrate, several GLHS interviewees believe clinical training, not gender, makes the difference in effective leaders. Spitzer reflects: "Clinical people are more territorial, and less business oriented—this applies to both males and females. Because of their functional specialty training, they are more task-oriented and less able to see the broad picture."

Also important is that when individuals diverge from the stereotypical behavior we expect, we frequently experience dissonance and even question their competence. These conflicts are not just external to the leader—they may also produce profound internal conflicts, as we shall explore in Chapters Four and Six.

Fully acknowledging the serious limitations of gender typing, we can proceed *with caution* to reflect on the leadership values we attribute to females or males in health care, or both. Not every female or male will exhibit these values. But these examples can enlighten our views of what leadership is and can become for both men and women.

Values, Gender, and Health Care Leadership

In the context of organizational or professional culture, values are embedded in the strategies and tactics through which the job gets done. When there is a contradiction between the stated values and the behaviors, we believe the behaviors. Values lead to management style and leadership preferences. Many are based in sex roles and sex role stereotypes, as we have seen.

For sociologists, "tribal" membership profoundly affects values and behavior within organizations (Neuhauser, 1988). And the most basic tribes are those of males and females. Even if men and women share the same values, Neuhauser suggests their thinking is organized differently, which results in different expressions of that thinking. In turn these tribal differences and expressed values can cause conflict.

Each tribe plays by its own values, or rules, which Neuhauser believes are different for the male and female tribes (Neuhauser, 1993). For example, competition and a pressure to perform drive males, she believes, and they generally attribute their success to their own ability and hard work. Perfectionism and pressure to please drive females, who generally attribute their success to luck and their failures to their own lack of ability. Women entrust more than men, expecting those around them to achieve the goals that have been laid out for them (Lipman-Blumen, 1996, p. 321).

It is important, too, to remain aware of the limits of these cultural biases, and their links to gender. GLHS contributor Alain Gauthier is a consultant to many health care organizations throughout the

United States and France, his country of origin. In his interview, he commented that the contrast between masculine and feminine qualities is greater in this country than in France. When Gauthier took a preference test as a twenty-one-year-old student at Stanford, he registered fairly high on "feminine qualities," whereas in France that score would have been "about average."

Although such contained views of group behavior are neither complete nor definitive, they do offer us a glimpse of the unconscious judgments and mores that drive groups of males and females in all organizations. When overlaid with the cultural standards of health care's professions and management, these dynamics become even more powerful forces.

Leadership as a Masculine Value

Leadership itself is a value-laden term, often suggesting aggression, competition, dominance, ambition, decisiveness—in other words, behavior often considered masculine and "better" (Klenke, 1996, p. 6).

Is the value of and drive toward competition a basic biological difference between males and females? Indeed, one view says that men want to conquer whereas women are ready to relate (Wilbur, 1996). Few would disagree that our cultural devotion to competition and opposition plays out in the corporate world at large. Of immediate concern is that the values we consider feminine have not had equal play in the decisions made at corporate tables, including many in health care.

Feminine Values

So-called feminine values of responsibility, connection, and inclusion are quite different from the traits of the competitive, rugged individual or lone hero model of leadership we have traditionally revered (Miller, 1997).

Implicit in the terms connection and inclusion are relationships. Traditionally, as one GLHS interviewee asserts, our society has assigned the principal tasks of social relationships to teachers, psychologists, social workers, and caregivers, who are primarily women. This GLHS contributor believes their "product" is not clear and that this nonquantifiable "softer" outcome is not highly valued by Americans. Linking these values with gender, she points out that the softer professions still receive low pay. "It is different for a surgeon, for example, who makes an incision—which can be regarded as a clear outcome," she says.

Contributor Patricia Cahill, J.D., adds that women see the world as made up of relationships, and they are not only better at building them but at dismantling them. She says, "Women are more honest— they are better at confronting hard questions in their professional relationships. Men will often back away from direct confrontations. They seem better able to live with nonresolution, even for years, as long as they don't get into major difficulty as a result of it."

Cooperation, too, is often considered a feminine value, and if it engenders trust it may lead to strategic affiliations and pooled resources. In successful alliances based on cooperation, trust is a huge factor. Leadership in these arrangements is usually accomplished by persuasion rather than through the hierarchical imperative of position or the power of formal authority.

Contributor Lawton R. Burns, whose extensive research on integrated health care systems was noted in Chapter One, has looked closely at the issue of trust in health care organizations. Burns believes that "women have certain positive attributes and certain negative attributes when it comes to trust. These are critical elements in the success of efforts to integrate. Among the positive things would be their strong communication abilities, their abilities to listen, and their interest and abilities in resolving conflict." He continues by saying that their negative traits can be perceived credibility and competence. (Further discussion of credibility and perceptions of competence are in Chapter Six.)

Another value considered central to the feminine spirit is caring. How does this play out for health care professionals? For nurses, a crucial value is caring for patients, often expressed as personal, hands-on attention. These nurses may respond angrily and passionately to financial constraints and resource changes they believe will affect staff levels and threaten patient care. This level of emotion is typical of tribal response when a key value is threatened (Neuhauser, 1993, p. 46).

How important are these tribal values to women's achievement of senior leadership roles in health care? They are quite significant. In a culture in which competition is highly valued, how does ambivalence in women and enthusiasm of men regarding competition play out in leadership? In a survey conducted by the American Management Association in the early 1990s, the researchers asked women if they had hesitated to pursue a promotion that would have placed them above the women they worked with. At least half of those who responded said yes (Duff, 1993, p. 46).

Values and Discord in Health Care Leadership

How do the sociological dynamics between males and females manifest in health care? A number of GLHS interviewees cite the penchant of their male colleagues for hierarchy, competition, and clear roles. According to Carol Gilligan's landmark work *In a Different Voice* (1982), women do not see the world in hierarchical terms, such as a ladder, but rather as a net or web of human connectedness. It is from these connections or "webs" that women build relationships. According to a number of researchers, interdependence can be difficult for men to achieve or strive for—because men need to exercise power over women.

One male who is a key leader in managed care and medical group practices observes that "women tend to do the right things for the right reasons—men tend to do the right things for the wrong reasons." Whatever the reasons, such cultural differences may account for this statement.

GLHS contributor Phyllis Kritek, Ph.D, R.N., an expert in conflict and negotiations in health care, says that men often base ethical decisions on principles, whereas women ground them in human needs and interests. "Both seem to think theirs is the only option," she continues, citing as an example the "do not resuscitate" order found in hospitals. From a male perspective, she says, such an order is a principle to which there are no exceptions. The female perspective, however, calls for trying to determine what the family wants. Kritek recommends a more effective approach for both men and women: take both perspectives into account. "What is more usual, however," according to Kritek, "is that Nurse Y will not offer her opinion because to her, Dr. X is in charge, he will always be in charge, and so he must be right. That strips her of accountability, as well as choices that might have been wiser."

The limitations imposed by ingrained gender roles are perhaps nowhere more evident than in the emergency room. As Spitzer notes, gender issues are often more pervasive here because of the intensity of the experience for all concerned. For the caregivers, the patients, and their families, this environment is crisis oriented and fast-paced, so gender may not at first appear to be an issue. But, as in other stressful situations, individuals often unconsciously revert to their early, learned responses. Spitzer observes, "Nurses for example often become more passive, which weakens their opportunity to be effective as collaborative partners with physicians and administration" (1997, p. 732).

The most poignant example of both ethical and practical dissonance is the story of a GLHS contributor who was CEO when his health system was at loggerheads with a contracting HMO customer. The HMO's male CEO severed the link between the two with fewer than thirty days' notice. This, says the contributor, could have had adverse effects on pregnant women in the last trimester, on high-risk pregnancies, and on patients needing dialysis, a procedure in which interpersonal relationships and trust play an important part. Public reaction to the HMO's action was negative. In fact, the press labeled it as a "'pissing contest' between the CEOs." He continues, "Had either CEO been female, a more humanistic approach on how to disconnect might have ensued."

Defining Leadership

We can now begin to understand the complexity of the issues embedded in the data and perceptions of gender's role in health care leadership. The summons of leadership for women presents an even greater challenge when mixed with the other prominent elements of this exploration: authority, expertise, power. All these ingredients mix together differently in every context, both inside and outside health care.

To move ahead, we will use the following as the best among many definitions of leadership: "Leadership is a role performed by an individual who exercises influence within a system in order to accomplish goals that flow from a vision and which are based on values" (Klenke, 1996, p. 12).

Leadership is also variously defined as behaviors, characteristics, theater, influence, power, authority, achieving objectives, and transformation—to name just a few of its meanings. These definitions take into account qualities of the leaders, traits of the followers, and leadership processes and outcomes.

The GLHS suggests that the leader as "guide of" and "participant with" people is the evolving form of leadership, as we move from the narrow notions of "command and control." In many instances, this form of shared leadership, or cocreation, is better suited to the future of many social institutions, including health care.

Enter the Lone Hero

But while this new leadership is evolving, we continue to experience the "lone hero" leadership paradigm and its effects. This is the "macho, self-reliant, clearly differentiated good guy in a world where the divisions are easy" (Noer, 1997, p. 164). These are the leaders we revere as heroes. We often put them on pedestals, making them larger than life. Traditionally, these heroes are leaders, and they are often health care experts, particularly physicians, as well.

Noer (pp. 164–166) observes that we usually like our heroes and our villains to be "strong, simple and clearly differentiated." We can blame or praise leaders for the clear roles they play, either well or poorly. We can also look to these leaders, rather than to ourselves, for accountability for the results we produce as a culture. Noer further notes that this is a process of delegation upward, implying that these problems can be fixed by these leaders—in other words, by someone else.

The type of leader often relied upon in the past, the "man with the answers," is simply not attainable nor even desirable in many situations today. The contexts in which we express our needs for leadership are simply too large and complex for this simplistic expectation. This is true for all major social institutions of our time: education, social services, and elected leadership at the national and local levels.

Health care is no exception. With the advent of managed care, the call for prudent medicine, the arrival of telemedicine, and the explosion of medical knowledge, medical experts can no longer afford to wait in their offices or in their classrooms for the patients and students to simply come to them. The labor- and knowledge-intensive nature of their work has shifted dramatically, as have the demands and sophistication of many consumers. Many health care purchasers are becoming more savvy about their options and better equipped to ask for and receive the medical interventions, complementary therapies, and preventive techniques they need. They are more likely to want to partner with their care teams to improve their own health. This has important implications for leaders and healers in the new order.

Being open to new calls on leadership, including the constant demand for appropriate resource allocation, while sharing one's mantle of expertise and power is not easy for any of us. It is especially hard for professionals. According to Gauthier, professionals are socialized to believe they should *know*, and when they don't or can't know it all, acknowledging that is difficult.

New Vantage Points on Traditional Leadership

To understand the opportunities of today's world, we must bring fresh perspectives to the shifting mandates of health care leadership and look beyond traditional management theory. For example, as chaos theory explains, the ordering of component parts is a repeating theme throughout nature. Fractals, as these natural repetitions are called, are present in all natural settings.

"Hierarchy" in nature is simply a framework for this order, and as such is not likely to disappear in nature or in organizations. Nor should it. Even in the most extreme examples of networked organizations there is hierarchy, according to Peter Senge, America's seminal thinker about learning organizations. In such organizations, it is a hierarchy of "guiding ideas." In these instances, the leaders exert their influence through "ideas they developed, which become embedded in the organization, not through on-going decision making" (Gibson, 1997, p. 141).

In traditional organizational hierarchies, however, we attach value and judgment to certain portions of the order at the expense of others. We may tacitly or blatantly consider some parts better than the others, and we bestow significance or power accordingly. Declaring one aspect more than, less than, better than, or worse than the others corrupts the real meaning of hierarchical order.

Riane Eisler (1987) describes traditional organizational hierarchies and the dissonance they can create for both women and men within them. As we value one part of an organized system more than the others, we soon move into domination of one part over another. It is this domination that for many creates conflict and discomfort. Referring to institutionalized domination that leads to debasement of other viewpoints, Eisler links this phenomenon specifically to male domination and female subordination.

Increasingly, however, organizations are finding that this polarity is neither necessary nor appropriate for solving the ever-complex situations they face. For example, nationally recognized management theorist Michael Hammer challenges this old yet persistent model of leadership by questioning the assumption that the most important work in organizational hierarchy is supervision. Indeed, he states that now "the real work, the craft, adding value, *is* the work, and this work is being performed by a team of professionals" (Gibson, 1997, p. 101). This has particular relevance to health care, where the "craft" is the work of not just medicine nor of any single group or profession. Rather, as the focus of health care changes to healing and wellness, we are called to embrace a more holistic or systemic approach. Treatment is not just aimed at the illness but at the causes of the illness and at the systems in which the illness flourishes.

Important to our understanding of attainment of senior leadership posts for women, Hammer notes, is that in the new model, professional advancement is not necessarily "up the ladder" but is often lateral, reflecting movement toward professional growth and achievement. Women (and men) may well be choosing this lateral path. Yet it is unlikely that this fully explains the findings of the recent ACHE study.

Unfortunately, many organizations' hierarchies have not changed to accommodate this new reality. However many or few of these old models exist today, those that remain can be rigid, comfortable, and safe while offering their leaders a large margin of control. In *Rethinking the Future*, Senge extends compassionate insight to those who want to remain in control: "Giving up control is very difficult, but it's virtually impossible if you have no idea of what you might be getting in its place" (Gibson, 1997, p. 140).

Eisler suggests an alternative to these clashes in world view and philosophy: a partnership model that equally values the viewpoints and contributions of multiple perspectives—in this case, those of both males and females. Through this model we can unleash actualization, rather than hierarchies that for many are unfavorable forms of power that lead to less than optimal results.

Ken Wilbur also renders a revised world view that is more appropriate for the work of today's organizations, health care included. In *A Brief History of Everything* he refers to "holons"—entities that are themselves whole and simultaneously part of yet another. He describes what happens when any particular element of the hierarchy, or holon, usurps its position when it wants to be "only a whole, and not also a part." The "natural and normal holarchy degenerates into a pathological or dominator holarchy. . . . We want to 'attack' these pathological hierarchies, not in order to get rid of hierarchy per se, but in order to allow the normal or natural hierarchy to emerge in its place and continue its healthy growth and development" (Wilbur, 1996, p. 27).

The partnership approach espoused by Eisler and the holarchy view proffered by Wilbur have many benefits. These are summarized well by David Noer (1997): "The conversations need to be about ways to live with snakes, ways to accept and accommodate their existence, as opposed to tales of how they are killed."

Health Care Leadership in the Knowledge Era

In the 21st century, health care will move well beyond the industrial era, through the service era, and into the knowledge era. Health care is both a service and an enterprise of scholarship. As an economic concern, it has focused in the main on providing medical care through centralizing and containing knowledge within the confines of its professions, prestigious institutions, and scholarly literature. According to GLHS contributor Wanda Jones, "the Internet will change all this. There are huge opportunities for health care in knowledge transfer, particularly in medical 'compliance', self healing, symptoms management and treatment choices."

But health care expertise, like that of other competency-based endeavors in the United States, has been based on the tradition of stockpiling information within the domains of its leading healers and executives and its most prestigious institutions. Economic theory attests to the traditional wisdom of this: creating scarcity creates value. Traditionally, the possession of specialized knowledge that few others have or know how to apply is treated with the highest regard and rewarded with the greatest tributes.

However, this perspective is very different from what John Sealy Brown, of Xerox's Palo Alto Research Center, calls for today in competency-based organizations. Such "communities of practice" offer an intriguing alternative for health care. "Communities of practice [form] the social fabric that emerges from sharing a task over a period of time," Brown says. "Core competencies live in these communities and surround them" (Gibson, 1997).

Bringing to life these new opportunities for inclusion requires different notions of leadership. Indeed, they require fundamentally different uses of expertise in which *all* members of the health care team can make vital, mutually valued contributions.

The next chapter brings to life the data and concepts presented in this chapter. It reviews the journeys of male and female GLHS contributors through the many worlds of health care stewardship and how they believe gender affected them along the way.

3

· ·

Experiencing Gender on the Job

From feeling constantly on guard around her male boss, to having to hire a man who would be paid more for the same job, to enjoying being the only woman in a room of men, GLHS contributors in this chapter describe their experiences moving through the gender-shadowed world of professional health care.

In this chapter I invite readers to compare these stories to their own and consider their own opinions about these questions:

- More than 90 percent of the study respondents believe gender plays a major role in health care leadership. How?

- How do we define effective leadership in health care for both women and men?

- How do male and female expressions of leadership differ, if they do?

- What happens when men or women don't conform to our expectations, even if stereotypical, about how leaders should conduct themselves?

The Effects of Gender on Leadership in Health Care

As we consider the viewpoints of the men and women who offered their opinions on this important issue, it is wise to consider the limitations of any qualitative study based on such perceptions. Even in controlled investigations, we cannot attach certain meaning to beliefs about gender or any *single* factor in an individual's array of unique characteristics.

As GLHS contributor Margaret Neale, Stanford University Graduate School of Business professor, offered in her interview: "If we are unable to isolate factors such as gender and professional training in research, how can we isolate these factors in everyday life?"

Still, such attempts are useful in understanding the part gender plays in the leadership experience. Even when we do not know how gender per se influences us, we may believe it is a significant consideration. A successful former chief executive officer of a major health system, Jane Neubauer, fifty, has had a fruitful career that includes experience as a staff nurse, professor, nurse manager, nurse director, vice president of nursing, and, currently, health care consultant. Of her leadership career, she says that it has always been complicated by "the fact that I am a nurse and a woman, so I was never sure whether reactions to me were related to the fact that I was a nurse, a woman, or neither."

Women Share Their Stories

Nearly 90 percent of female GLHS contributors said gender plays a major role in their stewardship efforts. The remainder said its role isn't major because they are already emphasizing both masculine and feminine traits or because other variables such as parenting or personality are more important.

The most striking quality of all the interviews was the sincere and personal reflection that accompanied them. Most contributors' propositions were straightforward in tone and language, with few if any bemoaning their fates. Many offered personal stories along with statements indicating they had never been asked these questions before.

Naturally, the comments and experiences are highly individual. Reaching universal understanding of the significance of this single issue is elusive, but several themes emerge:

Exceptional ability is assumed for some women because they have positioned themselves well. A female consultant in her late fifties and of national repute notes, "I was given credit early and excessively because so few have done this type of work. People believe I must have extraordinary abilities. This is not so—I just have competency, but in a woman, that has appeared to be something more."

A fifty-year-old human resources consultant has twenty-five-plus years of experience and a Ph.D. Previously a senior health care executive, she says that she deliberately positioned herself to serve corporations as an expert in leadership development and organization change: "Human resources is the only bastion of women in organizations. This is 'woman's work' . . . but I come at this from the point of view of strategy and organization. I am really combining male and female perspectives."

At times, some women are highly self-conscious as leaders. Gender becomes a greater factor in their exercise of leadership when they believe they are being challenged. Some second-guess themselves or change their styles to accommodate what they perceive as the prevailing "masculine" norm.

A female nurse in her mid-forties describes gender as a screen that goes up: "I don't feel this screen as much if I'm not feeling challenged. When I do feel a challenge, however, the red flag goes up. There is a power 'thing' going on—between doctors and nurses and males and females. It is hard to tease out what is what."

Another contributor shared the self-consciousness she experiences as she reports to a male for the first time in twenty-six years. "I am constantly on guard. I used to talk with my boss with stories and anecdotes, along with numbers. Now, I don't feel comfortable doing this. I worry that he will think that I can't make hard choices—that I'm just whining and complaining."

Some women are self-conscious about gender, but they enjoy it! Being the only female in a room is hardly a new experience for most women who participated in this study. Rather than feel uncomfortable about this, several women said they like it. They believe they are accorded more attention and courtesy than their male counterparts.

Many women believe gender affected their career choices. Many GLHS female contributors believe gender has placed serious constraints on those choices; fewer perceive no gender-related barriers at all. Naturally, the age of these women greatly affects their views. This topic will be explored in greater depth in Chapter Seven, but the following brief examples help us understand gender's influence early in these women's leadership lives.

A fifty-one-year-old female consultant with an impressive record of accomplishment speaks for many. She saw only two career choices: teaching and nursing. Like women her age in other fields, her ninth-grade Kudor Preference Test identified a strong aptitude for engineering, but it was not a popular choice for women at that time. She chose teaching. Eventually, she came to health care— albeit by a circuitous route.

Gender has not affected career choices "at all" for Leanne Kaiser Carlson, a thirty-six-year-old health care entrepreneur, consultant, and public speaker: "My situation is unusual—I never think about this." Gender wasn't emphasized as she was growing up, in part because she was raised without the concepts many people cast as masculine and feminine.

Dolores Clement, associate dean at the School of Allied Health Professions at the Medical College of Virginia campus of Virginia Commonwealth University, is about fifty. Clement says that gender hasn't affected her career choices either. She didn't realize that health care was so male dominated, but "this wouldn't have mattered. I had five brothers and four sisters—a huge family. I have always been comfortable with boys and men, and have usually had male friends and colleagues."

Some women avoid facing gender hurdles by mastering other obstacles that are easier to overcome. One contributor in a professional field enjoys considerable respect from her colleagues, but does not have a professional credential that many of them do. She often muses about whether she prefers that obstacle, which for her is a higher challenge, rather than gender difficulties. To her this may be "an avoidance of gender issues. I can transfer gender frustration into other blocks."

The gender-related leadership practices women have observed in other leaders influence their own strategies and career moves. One woman, about forty, practiced some years ago in a small consulting firm with both male and female bosses, whom she learned from with equal interest. Later, in a much larger firm that was "very male-dominated," she watched the women fail and command less money: "I watched my boss hire a guy who would make more money than I—yet I was supposed to train him. When I asked where my money (e.g., my equivalent compensation) was, I was told 'no one is irreplaceable.'" In response, she looked for an environment that was fair to women, and found one in which women comprise 40 percent of the partners. She adds, "My colleagues and I still have to 'remind the guys that we're there,' but before these issues were 'unmentionables.' Now I know I am highly regarded. I can speak up and not get 'squashed.'"

Carmen Nevarez, M.D., director of external relations for the Public Health Institute and faculty member at the School of Public Health at the University of California at Berkeley, considered herself very aware of the impact of gender on her life and career. "I selected [medicine] because it was the best vantage point from which to become a political leader. . . . Plus I had a natural interest in science. I recognized in Ben Casey, Dr. Kildare, and Marcus Welby the clear message that they were the authorities and were not to be questioned." Nevarez believes that authority gave her an edge in medicine, because "the fact that I am a physician always got me an extra point" that she would have lost "automatically" as a woman.

Women are concerned about the personal price of donning the male or dominant model of leadership. For Nevarez, this "edge" of authority brought a downside. Sometime during Nevarez' medical training, her mother told her that she was starting to become "like all those other doctors" (that is, men)—an "anti-women, anti-ordinary" person. "As angry as I was . . . I did reflect on this. I was very impressed with my mother—she was a fabulous feminist. I deliberately chose not to become overly masculine and bossy after this incident." Significantly, this awareness of perceptions about gender-related behaviors rather than personality-related behaviors enabled her to become more effective as a leader. "Before that, I was comfortable telling people with brains what to do and not to do," she says. "This wasn't effective. What was effective was to guide the group—like a sheep dog."

For some, gender's expression is directly related to age. A health care strategist in her fifties commented that for her gender is neither masculine nor feminine: "I have both qualities and as I get older, the more male qualities come out. I am blunter, I care more for ideas and achievement than consensus building and wading through lots of 'whining'—from men or women."

Some women make a deliberate choice to develop their masculine and feminine sides. Although only a few GLHS interviewees explicitly stated this, it is a key theme in Chapter Ten and worthy of mention here. A fifty-year-old woman said that it has been her conscious goal to "develop" both sides, despite some pressure to let the female side go. She describes herself as being "ornery enough and committed enough" to refuse. For her this is more than just theory. She applies this belief about balance while she reviews her institution's budgets, which she considers to be the ethical documents of the organization.

Men Share Their Stories

Fewer GLHS contributing males spoke to the question of gender's influence on career choice and leadership styles. However, a fifty-year-old physician with a distinguished career in policy, research, and academia comments that he is comfortable with a leadership style that is considered more feminine than masculine. He says that as his career has progressed, he prefers to emphasize team building, consensus, and collaboration. But, he adds, "I have also become quite comfortable being autocratic in the 20 percent of decisions where it's needed."

Another successful male states candidly that gender does have an impact for him: "There is an instinct—like Gregory Peck in *Twelve O'Clock High*—I am in charge, and I have the right answers." However, as the answers become less certain in today's changing environment, he must behave differently. "I have to learn to cope with ambiguity and step more easily out of this traditional role." One man in his mid-forties reports on the atmosphere when he took a senior executive position in a company in the mid-1990s. Women were a large portion of the workforce, yet the men had an attitude that "you can't tell 'em the truth." He adds, "Of course, this was behind closed doors."

What is Gender's Relationship to Effective Leadership?

In considering the link between leadership efficacy and gender, contributors nearly always appeared to speak from their experience and beliefs rather than theories. The GLH study posed the question, "Do you notice differences in effective leadership behaviors between male and female health care leaders? If so, what are they?" I asked each contributor to use her own definition of effectiveness and to explain what that was. I also asked respondents to focus more on gender comparisons of effectiveness than on other factors such as professional training.

Respondents' criteria for effectiveness fell into several categories:

1. Getting the job done
2. Getting the job done in a particular way—for example, looking good; not leaving things in disarray; getting results more

quickly and cheaply than competitors; being efficient or adding value; or succeeding in a balancing act, as by making policy, program, and numbers work together

3. Having the ability to move across disciplines, balance task and relationship, and balance masculine and feminine polarities—for example, assertion and receptivity, logic and intuition

4. Creating affiliations, partnerships, and collaboration

5. Having the staying power to remain in a powerful position in a major organization for (as an example) thirty years

6. Creating a harmonious workplace

7. Efficiently getting from point A to point B

Given these viewpoints, GLHS contributors' beliefs about gender's part in effectiveness fall into seven groupings.

On Authority and Positional Power

How women handle authority in others and themselves drew comments from several contributors. An organization's male president, for example, says that often his female colleagues are the ones who ask whether one of his statements is a decision or an opinion. They will also be more open about their personal needs, at times asking directly for permission to balance their lives as their personal circumstances require. He says this contrasts markedly with some of his male colleagues, who are more circumspect in their statements of need and personal travail.

Two women contrasted the way women handle positional power to that of men. Says one widely recognized executive, "Men tend to overdelegate, leaving people without clear direction and being too busy to clarify. Women are more accessible and clearer about what they expect, attempting to fit the understanding level to the individual." Another female executive says that "men are better able to delegate; women executives get more involved in the details." She then repeats an often-cited theme: "Men get other people to do it and take credit for it."

A physician with substantial management experience offers an observation that she realizes can be condemned as "politically incorrect": "I wonder whether women are less demanding of their subordinates. This is a two-edged sword: women welcome exceptional performance, yet they are much more tolerant of personal problems and difficulties. Therefore their units might accomplish less."

Several contributors cited female colleagues they consider to be overcontrolling. One states, "It takes a lot of energy to be so authoritarian, to figure out what everybody's job is and how to do it. You can get more done in this business, which is not one of widgets, with a collaborative, developmental style."

These comments reflect the limitations of gender typing, and the resistance women and men experience when those around them behave against type. (Chapter Four considers this problem and some possible solutions.)

On Success

Knowing the limits of loyalty is what distinguishes very successful female executives from those that are less so, according to GLHS contributor Peter Rabinowitz, a well-known recruiter of successful women health care leaders. "The most successful women know when to go, and they know the limits of being right, staying committed, and finishing the job," he says. Although these are values many women hold dear, he made clear that there can be too much of a good thing. Knowing when to push on, whether in a career position that's gone on too long or in a discussion that is no longer productive, is a key skill of highly accomplished women.

Another contributor, a female in her late forties, believes that because women are brought up to be pleasers, "It's hard for us to say no, and to walk away from a negotiation or task." She reported that she herself is learning to develop new boundaries to this end.

Kathryn E. Johnson, president and CEO of the Healthcare Forum in San Francisco, a key leadership resource for health care executives throughout the country, offers wisdom in this area. "It is always crucial to know that you can walk away—away from any deal, at any time. The minute we become too attached to a deal we're considering, we are too involved to be most effective in that negotiation."

Yet it is important to hold the notion of loyalty and its limits with care. Consider, for example, the woman at the health care insurance company who spent two years coaxing her superiors into implementing an innovative claims process that would save steps for providers and ultimately benefit patients. Her persistence paid off—particularly for the patients.

But too much loyalty or dedication to the job affects the everyday lives of female leaders. As a senior manager within a very large HMO observes, "When I was a nurse executive in a hospital, all of my counterparts were men. They always knew when the end of the day came." There is considerable cost to not knowing when to quit. Although admirable, women's dedication can have serious negative consequences for themselves and those around them. Carol Spain Woltring describes it well: "Women work very consistently and very hard. But with the intensity, dedication and long hours, they begin to feel it in their late forties and they begin to look at nonadministrative leadership roles in their fifties."

The relationship between vital leadership and regeneration is key, as these contributors attest.

On Taking Action

GLHS contributor Stephen Shortell, Ph.D., spoke for several interviewees who commented on male leaders they observe. Shortell, the Blue Cross Distinguished Professor of Health Policy and Management and professor of organizational behavior at the University of California at Berkeley, offered his observation with the caveat that exceptions certainly exist: "Male leaders I've observed appear to be better at making decisions more quickly."

Several people commented that men think through what they want as a matter of strategy, and once they've decided they don't let much interfere with taking action. When they focus their agenda on long-term results, they can afford to lose all sorts of short-term battles.

GLHS contributor Alain Gauthier noted that men's natural tendency is to be emissive, not receptive. In a recent seminar he facilitated, he was called on simply to "be there" for another person—a woman. He said it was very difficult for him to just stand by without trying to do something, a feeling that was shared by other men in the room. Gauthier believes that "leadership is like being a good midwife. Sometimes it *is* important to simply just 'be there.'" He says being empathetic and having a good balance of male and female energy is important, because otherwise people just react, particularly during chaotic times. "To just listen is very difficult for some people," he adds. "One must 'die', at least momentarily, as an expert and simply listen."

GLHS contributor Judy Miller, R.N., a Senior Fellow with the Institute for Healthcare Improvement in Boston, agrees: "For females, the process of questioning is the rule. Thomas Jefferson said 'the best thing to do is nothing.' For men, that is hard to do. They are hierarchical and decisions have to be made. Their bias for action is too great."

Although the bias for action attributed to many men often produces successful results, this approach is not always the best. According to a female consultant and former nurse executive in a major health system: "Men are narrow in their perceptions of what actions to take. For example, they do a great job of due diligence on the financial side, but they don't take the temperature of the organization."

On Nominal Leadership

One male GLHS contributor believes that becoming a nominal leader is easier for men than for women. He attributes this to social expectations of leadership that are narrow and gender specific: "In my city, a Yankee mill town, leaders have always been tough and autocratic. . . . A lack of toughness is seen as weakness, and this weakness is capitalized upon."

The application of hierarchy in organizations, particularly in the 20th century, is important, as we saw in Chapter Two. One male contributor says about formally assigned roles, "They afford emotional detachment at some level and that helps people to succeed and develop."

Yet a female contributor describes what she sees as a "male pecking order that is immutable and part of a highly inbred male culture. This makes men impervious to new information, and wary if 'it doesn't come from the captain of the team.' Often they will say 'I don't know what John wants'—referring to the head of the team." She calls this the empty-chair syndrome: "The guys feel a need for solidarity amongst themselves—and they borrow power from each other and from the boss. In my experience, if you give women the parameters, they will just get on with it."

On Sports

Not surprisingly, a number of women remarked that sports have greatly influenced male leadership styles. Molly Joel Coye says that for men, the social-athletic-business life is all "of a piece": "Men are effective at building a wide network of experiences that is not so crude a process as women think." Another highly placed female executive agrees: "Much of men's effectiveness is attached to their outside activities—such as golf, with its off-site decision making. I don't see women creating these same kinds of environments—our sports are more singular, such as running."

But such behavior is not always positive. One female talked about the darker side: "There is the perception that men play hardball—that their behavior is typically predatory and ruthless, and that they have no emotion around this . . . that they are playing some sort of political game. As a result, people will talk with them less, and less trust builds."

Another female noted that in her sphere the males all compete with each other, particularly at the governance level. She and another contributor commented on men's ability to "get away with [being aggressive]," noting too that in contracting negotiations, for example, it is acceptable to be aggressive. One points out the ever-present double bind: "If women are aggressive, however, they are called bitches."

On Consensus Building and Process

Many study participants cited the well-acknowledged female penchant for process and consensus building. Their comments highlight the strengths and challenges of these affinities. Douglas Scutchfield, M.D., for example, believes "Women are more likely to strive for consensus and they are less likely to be autocratic in approaches to problem solving. The theories suggest that the way women approach decision making is to assure that all have some, rather than basing these decisions on arbitrary views of merit or value. This has been my experience, as well."

Another man categorizes women as processing more and being better listeners than men. In leadership situations, "Women will look at both sides and get input. In one case of implementing a new block-surgery scheduling system, for example, a male decided to move forward in an autocratic manner. There was no buy-in, so there was a lot of reaction and 'acting out.' The second time around, the next leader, who was a woman, talked to people. By creating the climate for how to do the scheduling, this approach took hold and has been in place for two years."

An accomplished GLHS female contributor of many leadership "firsts" comments: "Women do process better and have a better understanding of the question. They do not leap to an answer or conclusion—there is an understanding of context at the bottom." In her leadership team at a major health care system, she does not "work with one man on my team that understands this process. Men are struggling more now and can't understand why we can't solve problems more quickly. Men have a harder time tolerating ambiguity."

Although acknowledging the value of consensus building, Joel Shalowitz, M.D., M.M., candidly expresses concern: "Many women have more of a collaborative style, reaching mutually agreeable outcomes. They lessen the tension and are good at minimizing conflict. But sometimes, this may occur at the expense of conflict and the best answer." (Chapter Five explores remedies to this drawback.)

Carol Spain Woltring interviewed thirty women in public health across the United States who have achieved notable results and acclaim. Commenting on the downside of a process orientation, she believes that "In general, shared leadership and dispersed power are not threatening to women. It is easier to embody these in their management and leadership. Sometimes, however, the women were viewed as being indecisive, so they are now sensitive to 'hanging out' too long. They are more successful as a result." She also drew an important distinction: "There is a difference between being a process person and being averse to action. When people involve themselves in process in order to avoid action on an issue, this essentially pushes the necessary action out indefinitely."

Summing Up

This chapter gives the reader a close look at the ways GLHS contributors view gender's role in leadership in health care, along with their beliefs about the nature of effective leadership and how female and male expressions of such leadership behaviors can differ.

Chapter Four offers readers a chance to put it all together—to consider the full dimensions of their gender-related experiences while sampling new perspectives and ideas for safer passage to greater effectiveness and success.

4

Coming to Terms with Gender's Impact

In a pilot study for the GLHS, a group of the highest-ranking women in the United States initially and without reservation acknowledged the often negative impact of gender on their lives as leaders in health care. A few months later, those same executives backpedaled on their earlier comments. Later many of them changed their minds yet again.

This chapter offers insight into these actions by examining the cultural forces that so powerfully exert themselves on even the most seasoned female leaders. As the final chapter in Part One, it summarizes the social vestiges that narrow females' chances for leadership success. It also briefly considers options for resolving these predicaments, laying the groundwork for the full-scale solutions discussed in Part Two.

Each dynamic here interacts closely with the others. But they are offered discretely so we can momentarily focus on each one. Options for resolving one dynamic can be enriched by also selecting from the other strategies here and in Part Two that best align with the reader's own needs and concerns.

These occurrences fall into three categories: Dynamics 1–8 are primarily about females, Dynamics 9–11 are about males, and Dynamics 12–17 are about both.

About Women

Dynamic One: Denial

Among some women there is a lack of openness about exploring gender issues and their effect on leadership success. A GLHS contributing female CEO comments that women "don't dwell on this issue. In fact, it is a nearly taboo subject." Why?

Denial may be present at many levels: within ourselves as individuals, within groups and organizations, and within professions. Reviewing this chapter's opening example of denial offers us a glimpse of its relationship to women already in roles of achievement. As part of my work as a principal and faculty member for the Center for Nursing Leadership in 1995, I conducted a small gender-related survey of twenty-five senior nurse executives throughout the country. (The center began as a joint effort sponsored by the Hill-Rom Corporation of Batesville, Indiana, along with the Network for Healthcare Management and the American Organization of Nurse Executives in Chicago.)

The nurses in the survey were collectively responsible for managing a large portion of the nation's health care resources, and they were viewed by many to be among the senior health care leaders in the United States. Written survey results mirrored the findings of the 1997 GLHS: more than 90 percent of the respondents declared that gender plays an important role in their professional lives and leadership roles. Yet several months later, when these same individuals were face to face at an educational retreat, most denied that gender plays such a role!

During that in-person meeting, several new influences were apparent. First, the group was face to face, whereas earlier they supplied their responses in writing. Second, the group had by then become a close-knit community. Finally, participants did not know a few newcomers who were present that evening. These factors surely came into play in the group's change of heart, but it is also possible that this dramatic about-face was a strong expression of denial. In fact, during the next twelve months most of these individuals reconsidered their statements, volunteering their updated viewpoints in writing, e-mail, and informal conversations. Their communications often cited denial as one explanation for their earlier behavior.

Opportunities for Change. As a psychological defense, denial helps us by protecting us. If denial does exist, it is important to consider what it may be preserving. This can be accomplished by exploring the topic and asking for feedback in a safe environment with trusted colleagues, family, or friends. Professional assistance is also an option.

In any case, it is useful to identify and work through whatever underlying denial there may be, so it no longer blocks options for greater effectiveness for women and the organizations that are committed to bring forth their talents.

One simple tool for exploring the presence of denial is to ask: How effective am I? Am I meeting the goals I have set for myself? Am I aware of circumstances beyond my control that may be influencing my answers to this question? What concern calls for me to look again? Are there trusted others who will help me understand how I can be more effective? How can I help the organization alter its dominant modes of action to accommodate talent expressed in different ways?

These and similar questions can be explored at many levels—within an individual, a team, or an organization. Key to the process is candid communication with individuals who can be believed. What we determine will prod important learning that will help us proceed to the next level of achievement and success.

Dynamic Two: Women, Boundaries, and Relationships

For many women, positive relationships are key to optimal job satisfaction. Yet when significant power differences are perceived among females within the same group, relationships can easily sour.

Horizontal violence describes the resulting clashes that can occur within groups who are of the same sex or in the same professional, cultural, or ethnic group. These disturbances to individual and group well-being and productivity can erupt because some in the group perceive themselves to be less valued than others who are more powerful (Roberts, 1983, pp. 21–30).

GLHS contributor Elaine Cohen, Ph.D., R.N., notes that this circumstance takes place when women physicians "go after" nurses—putting them down, calling them frustrated doctors, and the like. The same dynamics can also hold true between nurses. Cohen and others commented on how difficult camaraderie among nurses can be when this occurs.

Another aspect of this phenomenon is the importance of operating within strong personal and professional boundaries. Boundaries refer to the space between ourselves and other people that allows us to hold on to the definition of who we are. Without these limits, women can lose themselves and their objectivity along with their ability to function effectively as leaders.

To illustrate, we have seen that caring and connection are key values for many women. Whether inbred or cultural, a woman's orientation to relationship can weaken her boundaries when these values come into play. For example, when should a female challenge a friend and colleague's actions rather than simply invite reflection on their appropriateness? If a woman feels strongly about such actions yet does not share her concern in any form, she fails to draw the line and stand up for her beliefs. She may engage in this behavior with both men and women, off and on the job. In so doing, she contributes to her own discomfort and does not develop integrity—a key personal skill upon which effective leadership is based.

Georgetown University sociolinguist Deborah Tannen has written frequently about differences in the ways men and women express themselves and understand one another. Tannen (1990) believes that women don't want to appear better than other women because this violates their egalitarian sensibilities. What is important to women, she contends, is connection and similarity rather than difference.

When we couple these factors with embedded perceptions and beliefs about power and the subconscious notion that if I win you lose, we can better understand the profound ambivalence some women have about leadership advancement. A GLHS contributing female consultant says it well: "Solidarity among women is only sustained if no one else in the group gets ahead."

Women's underlying preferences for symmetry can deeply affect their career decisions. Some women may emphasize maintaining a friendship over making a career move or accepting a promotion. Friendship and bonding for women can be based on sameness, and when one breaks that connection what will happen to the friendship? This is a very real concern for women as leaders, as we saw in Chapter Two in the survey conducted by the American Management Association.

This bias toward sameness, which can also be interpreted as loyalty, prompted one GLHS interviewee to say: "To the extent that we are preoccupied with each other negatively, then we are losing the war." This cuts both ways—when we are preoccupied with symmetry and fairness, there can also be a reluctance to move beyond these friendships, even when they no longer serve the work at hand.

For example, a senior executive described as "frustrating and depressing" the experience of letting another female manager go because she did not fit within the organizational structure. "This was a woman on my team whose behavior embarrassed me, and I put up with it a lot longer than I would have with a man," she says. "The woman had a family history that was not positive, and this affected how she interacted with her staff. She was provided with counseling, testing, and other resources, all at the organization's expense. . . . she was simply unable to change the behaviors that were required."

Opportunities for Change. For some, developing the capacity to set and keep boundaries is lifelong work. Such women may want to seek professional help and are well advised to pursue training in being assertive.

Anyone who is concerned about her reduced effectiveness today can acquire new tools that will immediately help her create more viable and satisfying work relationships. Numerous study contributors offer advice, techniques, and tips throughout Part Two that can be tailored to the personal needs of each reader so she may enhance her portfolio of skills while developing a growing sense of autonomy and power.

Building such skills starts with two key underlying notions:

- Perceived power differences between others and ourselves does not equal differences in our value. Individuals, departments, and organizations who mutually value the gifts of all members of the team, regardless of their place in the hierarchy, engender mutual respect within groups and between individuals.

- Although it is tempting to sweep loose boundaries and their effects under the table, doing so perpetuates abuses of relationships, which eventually render these relationships untenable. In an atmosphere of trust, it is important to air concerns about these behaviors before they reach this stage and to explore mutually beneficial solutions.

Dynamic Three: Low Self-Esteem

For some women, low self-esteem and the belief that their efforts are less than significant can affect their aspirations and others' perceptions of their abilities.

Two findings raise the possibility that this is true for some women in health care. The first, which surfaced in the 1990 ACHE study, concluded that the aspirations of women to leadership roles are significantly lower than those of males.

The second was brought forward by GLHS contributor Diane Littlefield, M.P.H., program director of the Women's Health Leadership Program in Sacramento, California, a developmental program designed for community health leaders throughout the state. "A lot of women in positions of responsibility do not see themselves as leaders," she says. "I hear a common theme among them: they will not apply for this program because they don't see themselves as eligible." She adds that this phenomenon does not appear to be related to age.

A number of other GLHS contributors also commented on the impact of low self-esteem among women in health care settings. To set the stage, consider the concept of "learned helplessness," introduced by author Nicky Marone. Learned helplessness, according to Marone, "is a self-defeating condition which keeps many women from confronting risk and benefiting from opportunity. It ensnares a woman in a tangled web of paralyzing beliefs, emotions, and behaviors. She consistently doubts herself even when she performs at consistently high levels. . . . Criticism can immobilize her" (Duff, 1993, p. 82).

One GLHS contributor who is a nursing leader says that as a leader, she frequently reflects on this key question: "Do nurses come to us with poor self-esteem or do we create it in them?" She sees the significance of increasing nurses' self-esteem so that they can competently participate in decision making, adding, "This is a critical gender issue for the future success of health care organizations."

The glass ceiling in health care was the focus of the Institute for Healthcare Improvement's Fall 1995 newsletter, *Quality Connection.* The institute assembled a panel of accomplished leaders and asked what barriers they anticipated as women move ahead. Panel member Gayle Capozzalo replied that the first barriers were internal: "Above all, [the barrier is] self-esteem or confidence. Studies show that women feel they have to know at least 75 percent of a job before they are even willing to apply for it, while men don't even feel they have to know 50 percent" (*Quality Connection,* 1995).

Low self-esteem can seriously affect a leader's effectiveness, which can further play itself out in perceptions of trustworthiness. Although Lawton R. Burns, Ph.D., whose work on trust, organizational affiliations, and leadership was discussed in Chapter Two, did not link these factors to self-confidence, we can conjecture that there may be a relationship. Burns notes: "If women are not perceived as able to do the job or as having enough time to commit to 'delivering the goods,' they will be viewed as less effective, and therefore, less trustworthy." (Chapter Six offers further evidence of this concern in communication, along with specific skills to offset it.)

Most women and men who are familiar with low self-esteem will recognize its important corollary: low self-trust. Self-trust is crucial to the internal "navigation system" that guides the leadership course. For example, one female GLHS contributor offered her view of what happens when women are confronted, directly or indirectly, by a lack of support from others: "We get hooked because we don't trust ourselves to 'just do it'—in other words, to take action. We have forgotten how to trust our instincts."

Opportunities for Change. Women who suffer from feelings of low self-worth are well advised to seek feedback and counsel of those closest to them. Some will be best served by seeking professional guidance, much as those who have difficulty setting limits. In both cases, exploring the causes of low self-esteem provides enormous relief and freedom.

Equally important, individuals who wish to bolster their self-esteem are well served by enhancing their capacities and skills—then they have no cause for less than full confidence. Honoring the principles of mutual valuing serves organizations well, too. In so doing, they will contribute to the self-confidence of their team members and reap the benefits of more productive organizational contributors.

Dynamic Four: Women Can Overdo It

We have seen the importance of setting limits on loyalty, whether to employees, to the tasks that remain at the end of the day, or to staying in a job when it is no longer the best choice. At the same time,

some women don't set limits on their personal sacrifices—they simply do too much. There is an ironic, destructive, and self-perpetuating cycle to all this "doing." GLHS contributor Dolores Clement, Ph.D., says it well: "Women have a hard time delegating and letting go so they can self-renew. They need to put people around them and trust that things will be there when they return." She adds an important, honest assessment of the true nature of most health care leaders' work: "Most of health care is not life or death. Yet, as women, we think we have to deal with everything." (Chapter Eight discusses the tolls so much activity takes on women. It also offers options for reducing commitments and regenerating for maximum productivity and enjoyment.)

Another female GLHS contributor adds insight into the measure of women's dedication: "Women tend to do their jobs and tasks by themselves. They work harder to achieve the expected, and often do more than expected." Are we to conclude that the female's proclivity to do too much derives from just her own sense of excellence? Although that may be part of the explanation, several contributors think differently. "Women executives constantly feel the pressure to prove themselves," says one.

The importance of this dynamic is evident not just in what women do. Many women bring equal determination to holding sway with their beliefs and values. This is surely an asset in many instances, but there are times when dogged insistence does not serve their goals, others on the team, or themselves. One male GLHS contributor who works with many successful female leaders sees this happening in some women, and he has concern. "They always need to be right, and it's a trap," he says. "Women are too attached to the outcome. They take a high moral ground—rather than revering efficacy." He observes that this is "evidence of women's focus on their own needs, rather than the needs of the situation."

Opportunities for Change. A key skill that leaders bring to each situation is discernment. When women are tempted to remain overly loyal to a point of view or an issue about which they feel strongly, they will benefit by considering the wisdom of their commitment through moments of reflection. This is particularly so when their internal navigational systems such as intuition are telling them to pursue a different course. Asks one male contributor who works with many successful women: "Is she interested in being right or is she interested in being relevant?" There are times when being right *is* being relevant—and there are also times when sticking to a particular position no longer serves current needs.

Women who simply do too much come by this habit through noble intentions and a strong cultural heritage that exists both inside and outside health care. Yet the importance of balance in maintaining one's own spirit and health, and her value to the team, is well documented. Most women know this, but they still find it difficult to cut back and refocus their efforts on the points of greatest impact. They are sure to benefit if they watch or directly ask for guidance from women and men who excel at managing their time in balanced and effective ways.

Dynamic Five: Taking It Personally

Loyalty can also play itself out for female leaders through attachment to emotions such as grudges. One female observer says that women personalize and don't get over their losses easily: "Women don't lose as gracefully as men. They can carry the hurt longer than men. I've known women who have held onto resentments for years."

"Taking it personally"—*it* being criticism or a message perceived as an attack on a woman as an individual—is a problem for many working women, according to about a half-dozen GLHS contributors as well as outside researchers. A female nurse executive who has practiced in various clinical and academic settings recently moved to a new environment with mostly women. In making this decision, she stated that she had to think about "working with all females. I like being direct and I notice that men do not 'take it personally.' Men can 'bracket'—and not hold a grudge." She adds that this inability to critique themselves or each other can preclude women from seeking or hearing feedback that will enhance their professional growth.

Opportunities for Change. Many women will do well to honor yet manage their emotions. Showing regard for emotions helps keep them in check, leaving women free to respond and engage with others without being personally engulfed. In so doing, they also bolster their self-esteem and deepen their limit-setting abilities.

Dynamic Six: Ambivalence About Power

Throughout the earlier chapters, we have seen many examples in which ambivalence about power is at play. Two instances illustrate this all too well: the women who do not wish to move to positions of greater responsibility as documented in the GLHS and the 1995 ACHE study, and the ways in which women and men act negatively by employing horizontal violence toward those whom they consider less powerful.

Power as a value causes difficulty for many women in this society. Yet at its root, power is a gender-free term that means the ability to influence and accomplish. In this culture, however, it is often revered as individual achievement (that lone hero model again) and displayed as the person in power being superior to others. Our beliefs about power are frequently based on either-or assumptions suggesting that one person, discipline, organization, or system is better than, greater than, and has "more" than another. Simply stated, this philosophy is "some win; others lose."

Adding to some women's ambivalence about power are perceptions that having power is being selfish or unfair to others. Such conflict can create profound feelings of discomfort in women, as well as men.

Opportunities for Change. Many women fare better in environments that are based on cocreation, cooperation, and collaboration. When these qualities are present in any context in which women and men work together, they can unite them in strength. In turn, this is beneficial to the organizations of which they are a part.

Women who are in positions of influence can help create these settings for the benefit of other women, as well as men who are also interested working together more effectively. (Chapter Five explores power in greater detail.)

Dynamic Seven: Women Can Undermine Their Own Effectiveness

In understanding how women can unconsciously sabotage their own goals, we learn by considering the significant differences in the socialization processes between one health profession and another. One GLHS contributor, a male who is highly experienced with both physicians and nurse leaders, comments, "Doctors have been bred to be dominant by the medical culture, and the reverse isn't true for women in nursing. The result is that nurses play a role in their own difficulty by not speaking up. Instead, they are often passive-aggressive." Another study contributor commented similarly, adding that some nurses do transcend this. But in his experience, "Many will spend a quarter of a given interaction 'getting back.' This is not helpful."

Opportunities for Change. Here we see a vivid example of several dynamics acting together: gender, physician and nursing culture, and the degree to which experiences in our past color our beliefs about what is occurring today. The guidance of the GLHS contributors is useful here too as we move to mutual valuing, greater self-esteem, more assertive behavior, and creating stronger boundaries between others and ourselves. All of these practices will enhance our abilities to act from strength. Women who hone these skills along with their competence can *act as if* their worlds will respect these strengths. In so doing, they *will in fact* become more effective. If they are not respected in their organizations after developing these qualities, they will do well to change their environments to better suit their needs, beliefs, strengths, and aspirations.

Dynamic Eight: Many Men Do Understand

A female contributor who works closely with men says that men are tired of being told they don't understand women. She offers an important perspective: "In health care culture, we are in a period of transformation—to espouse that men do not appreciate women is a throwback to old confrontational tactics. Females who say this do not have any recognition of how men are attempting to change." Her viewpoint resonates closely with the demeanor, willingness, and thoughtfulness exhibited by the men who participated in the GLHS.

About Men

Dynamic Nine: Privilege Deprivation

The term *privilege deprivation* is used to describe the experience of many men in today's corporate environments. This psychological dynamic comes into play when a shift occurs such as white women and people of color moving into positions held previously just by white males (Briles, 1996, p. 41).

Accustomed to being at the center of things, the white male today is often just one more contender for the spotlight and may believe he is at a disadvantage. Rosener describes this phenomenon as the loss of the "knapsack of privilege." In interviews with men in a variety of fields, she found that many men feel they are under attack and are not sure why. As they described their working relationships with women, these men reported three major issues of concern: "loss of power and control; loss of male identity and self-esteem, and increasing discomfort" (Rosener, 1995, pp. 84–100).

Opportunities for Change. Deep personal change is difficult for men and for women. Offering understanding as we strive for new relationships within ourselves and with others permits us to be compassionate rather than to place blame.

As women and men move through the challenges presented by gender's role in the changing mandates of leadership, we can acknowledge that it *is* a difficult time for those who are used to being considered, if not selected, for the most senior posts. Not only have these men been groomed for the top jobs, but they also have well-stoked expectations that they will have them. Such anxieties are compounded if related expectations are uprooted too. Older physicians, for example, are often angry and unhappy as they believe their places at the top of the economic heap are threatened by new economic realities.

Dynamic Ten: Sexual Static

Sexual static is Rosener's (1995) term for what men and women can experience when working in new ways with one another. For men, as described in Chapter Two, this static can cause unconscious discomfort. When Rosener asked how men feel about *supervising* women, they say they have no problem. When working with women as *peers*, they describe this as a new experience, one in which they may perceive a loss of control and power. When *competing* with women, they feel anxiety, which Rosener found is exaggerated in an atmosphere of corporate consolidation, including downsizing in health care. Rosener was unable to gather much information about men working *for* a woman, but what she did attain suggests two distinct reactions: men either like it or they don't.

Men who don't like the experience report feelings of confusion, irritation, anger, anxiety, tension, and devaluation. Men who say they are comfortable working with women have these qualities (Rosener, 1995, pp. 98, 100):

- They are secure in their positions.

- They have high self-esteem.

- They often have professional wives or daughters who are pursuing careers.

Opportunities for Change. The previously cited remedies for improved self-esteem, along with a renewed vision of health care leadership, will prove invaluable to men who feel threatened. As advised earlier in this chapter, personal counseling or discussions with trusted friends, family, colleagues, and trained individuals can also help alleviate these real concerns and feelings of loss.

Many men *consciously* welcome women who are assuming multiple roles of responsibility, technical support, and leadership at all levels of society in the United States. Sometimes, however, they may *unconsciously* revert to interacting with their female colleagues as mothers, daughters, wives, or even sexual partners—even though sexual harassment concerns are prominent in most men's consciousness today. Said another way, both men and women are freed when men deliberately develop new habits of seeing and interacting with women beyond their traditionally assigned sexual roles.

At the same time, we must encourage a full range of leadership expression for both men and women. As men become more free to air vulnerabilities and emotions without losing the respect of others, and as women don more masculine leadership behaviors without reprise from their colleagues, both will be more balanced. They will also bring new talents to bear as leadership roles evolve to accommodate the changing needs of health care populations and organizations.

Dynamic Eleven: Inbred Male Culture and Closed Organizational Climates

Several female GLHS contributors believe at least some men lack respect for the significance of organizational climate. As one contributor states, "Many men recognize 'business' achievement only. This means they don't acknowledge innovations, nor do they recognize patient approval and support. They simply don't know how to value them." A well-traveled male executive echoed this perspective. He adds that "an over-emphasis on numbers and an under-emphasis on organizational culture is a sure recipe for failure."

In a related theme, several other contributors cast the male culture in health care as highly inbred, which can make men impervious to new information. This is particularly true if the new information "doesn't come from the captain of the team." One GLHS participant, a consultant, has seen well-positioned men defer to their absent leader on a number of occasions. This relates to the "empty-chair syndrome" described in Chapter Three, and reflects the need for solidarity if not equality among men, as well as the ability to borrow power from one another.

Opportunities for Change. Male culture has many benefits from which women can learn to augment their own skills. For example, a number of female GLHS contributors believe that men network for specific career advancement, whereas women network for connection and friendship—regardless of where these relationships may lead professionally. But women can network for jobs too—while still cultivating their friendships. This is just one example of the benefits male and female cultural traditions can offer members of both sexes.

Males and females who wish to work in atmospheres of equality and openness are always well served by focusing on their mutual objectives while continually adjusting their dialogue to achieve them. Doing this takes the conversation between men and women away from differences in style that may never be resolved, and toward common aims that hold great promise for mutual success.

About Women and Men

Dynamic Twelve: We "Do" Gender Unconsciously

In *The Mismeasure of Women*, Carl Tavris (1993) posits that both males and females screen for gender unconsciously. In this process, we adjust our attitudes and behaviors depending on the sex of the person we are working with. Chapter Six, which focuses on communication, offers dramatic evidence of this phenomenon.

The power and impact of the masculine model of leadership pervades our daily interactions. When we are not aware of the salience of this embedded leadership archetype, we are left with stereotypes, unspoken concerns about effectiveness, and limited choices for leadership expression by both men and women. These cultural artifacts persist despite increasing belief that the best leaders draw from a combination of male and female traits.

Opportunities for Change. Men and women in health care can greatly benefit from heightening their awareness of their own unconscious gender-typing habits. Developing new sensitivity is freeing to all on the leadership continuum. All receive more latitude as a result of broadened thinking, particularly when senior leaders offer themselves as models. Health care organizations recoup in numerous ways, such as higher morale, increased creativity, and greater accountability.

Dynamic Thirteen: The 10 Percent Factor

Those who number fewer than 10 percent within a larger dominant group find their minority status to be a powerful determinant of their behavior and attitudes (Kanter, 1977, pp. 222–230). This fact, when coupled with the masculine version of leadership to which our culture is accustomed, strongly predisposes some individuals to adopt leadership behaviors we consider masculine.

A GLHS contributor who has worked closely with many senior female leaders observes just this phenomenon in health care: "We are at the crossroads in this country for leadership. The women who make it tend to be clones, or caricatures of men. The percentage of women in these positions is a little better now, but if you look at the excruciating selection criteria, the women who don't know how to play better than men, don't make it." The cost, says this contributor, is an imbalance of valued leadership characteristics: "When these women do make it, they may be more political, and more destructive than most men." Can women measure up if the standards we hold for these leaders are based on only the masculine model of leadership?

Opportunities for Change. Increasing the number of women in senior roles creates new opportunity for balance among male and female ways of being and doing. With care, women who have overemphasized male behaviors can nurture the feminine approaches they have deemphasized or even lost.

Dynamic Fourteen: Either-Or Thinking

Either-or thinking epitomizes the dichotomous world view that only two options exist, rather than a range of alternatives. This belief system produces polarities of all types: good versus bad, right versus wrong, me versus you, us versus them, strong versus weak, passive versus aggressive. On some occasions these black-and-white descriptors are appropriate, but in most instances they are not.

How relevant is either-or reasoning to health care? According to GLHS contributor and consultant Alain Gauthier, it exacts a significant price: "In my discussions of strategies with senior health care leaders, I can hear the polarities. 'Mission *or* business.'" The challenge, according to Gauthier, is to find the "both/and"—meaning engaging in sound business practice while also accomplishing the organization's mission. Although intellectually, groups often buy the *concept* of both-and, finding the right *operational* answers within that context is not easy.

Even more limiting than either-or thinking is our society's proclivity to revere the single best answer. Although the simplicity and elegance of one right answer is appealing, it is so confining as to be blinding. We are simply unable to see, let alone welcome, other options for the myriad and complex challenges faced everyday in health care's workplace. Rosener (1995, p. 24) offers relevant insight on the role that this dynamic plays in gender obstacles for women: "The barriers women face in the workplace probably have more to do with the one-best model than with their aptitudes and preferences."

Opportunities for Change. No one way is the *right* way. According to the GLHS contributors, the best leaders identify the *optimal* route to today's highest priority goals while remaining flexible enough to receive new information and to make course corrections as they are needed.

To find the best solutions to current challenges, effective leaders invite diverse and learned opinions and create opportunities for managed discord. They also embrace the nondual perspective, which honors and respects differences, while stimulating multiple options when time permits.

In the context of gender, considerable tension often exists between the feminine value of caring and the masculine value of business, as we have seen. As a consultant, Gauthier finds that "the 'solution' is to articulate very clear guiding principles that everyone in the organization can internalize." (Chapter Five provides strategies for and examples of managing discord.)

Dynamic Fifteen: Acknowledging the Dark Side

One of the most compelling reasons to honestly assess and respect who we are in our fullness—including those aspects we do not like—is that these powerful forces will make themselves known to us and to others in some way. Organization behavior experts David Noer (1996) and William Bridges (1980) both strongly encourage honoring the need to grieve, for example, when organizational transition takes its many tolls. In fact, there is business value to grieving and venting.

When left untended, these normal human emotions get stashed in a kind of invisible backpack—one we lug around with us. The danger of these, according to Noer, is that "they get too heavy, wear down the bearer . . . [and] the pebble that gets put in by an innocent, causes the burden to become too severe, and there is an outburst" (1996, p. 60).

GLHS contributor and author Phyllis Kritek offers an example of this dynamic when applied to health care. Figure 4.1 depicts a victim-perpetrator-rescuer cycle that can easily take hold when such unacknowledged burdens become too heavy. Women or men can enter the triangle at any point, begin a circle of dysfunctional behavior, and create an unruly, unproductive cycle for all involved. The behaviors may be subtle, but their presence is felt by all those in the cycle—regardless of whether they are conscious of them. Although the following example is harsh, Kritek instructs us on the

Figure 4.1. Victim-Perpetrator-Rescuer Cycle.

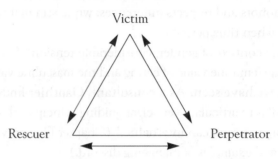

Published with permission from Phyllis Kritek, Ph.D., R.N., Center for Nursing Leadership, October 1997.

power of this dynamic: "I watch [some women] act as victims rather than liberated women or equals with men. They will do this until they burst out and display anger and rage out of proportion to the issue. They will also express solidarity with each other rather than seeking autonomy as grown women with the right to speak and act on their own behalf."

Opportunities for Change. Noer's vivid description of "rocks in our packs" suggests an elegant and simple solution: drop the rocks. If anger and aggression are appropriate, they may be employed to their full measure of effectiveness. But when they do not serve, their expressions are barriers to solutions—impediments to those who bear their weight while unconsciously inflicting it on others.

Dynamic Sixteen: Habits of Thought

Habits of thought, or "pulls of the groove," greatly limit our openness to emerging paths of leadership. Noted author and leadership authority Joseph Jaworski calls these pernicious default behaviors "traps": "Traps cause a regression to old ways of thinking and acting, thus hindering . . . the unfolding generative process. These snares emit a powerful pull, and yet when they are deeply examined, there is little substance to them" (1996, p. 21). The result: we don't have access to the full range of our talents and thus our many capacities to manage effectively.

Adaptation to the professional and social norms in health care can enshroud its leaders in an insidious barrier that blocks awareness, growth, and effectiveness. Unconscious of this block, we become increasingly insular yet comfortable with our way of handling challenges. At the same time, we may inadvertently develop more and more narrow mind-sets. A GLHS contributing consultant who has worked with many hospital administrators over the years describes one such situation: "If I could change anything, it would be to have executives rise above their locked-in, mutually dysfunctional relationships with the medical staff to care more and work more for the population they are serving."

Health care culture's deep roots are not always life-giving or life-helping, particularly when professionals must work with other disciplines to accomplish their mutual goals. The professions often operate much as real clans do, perpetuating the values, dialects, history, educational standards, and preferences of the group. Health care is filled with tribes—usually called disciplines—including those in this short list of examples:

- Primary care physicians and specialists

- Clinically trained and nonclinically trained workers

- Practicing clinicians and clinically trained leaders who no longer practice

- Local caregivers and system-based management personnel

- Professional and support staff

Opportunities for Change. The growing call for care that is coordinated across a continuum of services, institutions, and the community requires cooperation among all providers. We simply can no longer afford to operate from the narrow confines of one or the other viewpoint or vested interest. Patients deserve coordinated health care resources, payers demand economy, and institutions must generate cooperative strategies in order to provide quality care while exercising economic prudence.

Most health care executives know and live with these truths each day. But implementing these mandates is challenging. We need to break through the barriers caused by habit, socialization, and even preference. Women and men need to become comfortable with the discomfort that accompanies working with those with different belief systems.

The way is made far easier with the knowledge that most individuals in health care are committed to common values and a common goal—greater service and care for those in need. No single leader or professional can achieve this goal without greater, sincere reliance on others on the team. This can only be achieved if we embrace alternative perspectives while focusing on the best interests of the patient and consumer. (As noted, Chapter Five offers suggestions for managing conflicts and negotiating difference.)

Finally, health care leaders who regularly renew themselves personally and professionally while encouraging it in others go a long way toward relaxing the grip of unproductive habits. They aren't as likely to default to ingrained learned behaviors that simply don't serve.

Summing Up

This concludes Part One, which examines key factors that strongly influence gender and leadership in health care. The chapters in Part Two explore specific techniques, tips, and solutions for moving through and beyond these factors. To start, Chapter Five discusses and defuses unwanted aspects of gender's role in conflict, negotiation, and power.

Part II

Antidotes for Effectiveness

5

Antidote 1: Defusing Gender's Role in Conflict, Negotiations, and Power

To understand the relationship of gender to conflict, negotiating, and power in health care leadership, this chapter examines the following:

1. Male and female approaches to disagreements, negotiations, and risk-taking in leadership situations

2. Achieving common aims by promoting and managing differences

3. New models of power and GLHS contributors' experiences with implementing them

Gender's Role in Disagreements, Negotiations, and Risk Taking

Readers may find familiar the idea that women negotiate for results different from those of their male counterparts—women negotiate for closeness and men negotiate for position. This difference affects their abilities to manage conflict and negotiate, according to GLHS contributor and researcher Lawton R. Burns. He concludes that women are better than men at these two processes, in part because of their communication skills. "Men are more likely to want to sweep problems under the rug, quickly admit they were wrong—if they were—and move on because they are more action and future-oriented," he says. "Women, on the other hand, want to talk about it and sift through it." Several other male GLHS contributors echoed his statements, and a female contributor—a highly successful CEO of a national organization—added her view of conflict at the leadership table: "I have a forthright, direct approach to getting issues on the table for resolution. I feel it is tough for men to do this."

Not all women are able to be straightforward in conflict-ridden environments. Psychologist and author Joan Borysenko (1996) says about such female reticence, "One of the unspoken rules of adult feminine behavior is that women must buffer strife." This belief suggests that lifelong conflicts between being "nice" versus being "selfish" create a devil's dilemma for women. Adds Borysenko, "If a woman makes the choice in favor of other people, she . . . suffers a loss of self. . . ." With such cultural messages encouraging women to be "nice," it is little wonder that women are often not able to speak on their own behalf when conflicts emerge as they go about their work.

Some researchers purport that two different types of negotiating styles come into play in health care. "Claimers" are negotiators who grab what they can, thrive on conquest and winning, and play a zero-sum game. "Creators" forge connections among parties and a sense of shared destiny. When a claimer and a creator negotiate, however, the creator tends to come out the loser (Marcus and others, 1995). These modes might easily fit the gender-based stereotypes considered thus far—claiming is the masculine style, and the creator style matches what is considered feminine.

But is there a feminine decision-making style? Decision making is still an area in which the male model dominates. The styles we consider masculine, according to Marcus and others (1995), are "quick, assertive, and the decision is made with apparent confidence. We still look to this model as being the 'best.' Men tend to be more analytical, extracting what they consider to be essential."

If there were a style to feminine decision making, it might be called "consultative," a process driven by consensus building. Those whose expectations of decision making are based on the male model may view the female who gathers opinions, data, and takes her time as less than equally competent.

Deborah Tannen (1994) also purports that two different communication styles exist in negotiating, and both are useful in considering male and female preferences. With the "inside-out" style, an individual states what is wanted, starting "inside" and working her way out, such as by saying, "I'd like to see the two departments merge for greater efficiency and cost savings. What do you think?" In this case, others who have a different preference are expected to express that preference. In the "outside-in" style, the speaker may ask, "What would you like to do?" Both strategies work equally well—unless the expectations regarding negotiations and communications styles are different. Then the outside-in style may be perceived as vague, particularly if the viewer is considering the question with an unconscious bias for the inside-out strategy.

Health care leaders concerned about successfully negotiating in atmospheres of silent and unconscious judgments on effectiveness can improve their chances for success in two ways:

- By stating explicitly what process they are using. For example, if a woman believes her group shares her aim, she may say that, for a limited time, she is asking others' opinions to improve their chances of meeting a mutual goal.

- When called for, making decisions in a straightforward manner even when it does not feel comfortable. The ability to move from one's dominant mode of action to another less familiar approach may be difficult, particularly at first. But gaining facility with *all* the tools of leadership effectiveness, rather than only those that are most comfortable, is an important skill for those who aspire to the highest levels of leadership. (Chapter Ten offers a broader view of this concept.)

Other Considerations About Decision-Making and Negotiating Differences

How real are these perceived differences between men and women negotiators? According to GLHS contributor, Stanford professor, and expert on negotiations Margaret Neale, real differences do not exist *after the negotiations are under way.* She cites a small body of research conducted in the 1960s that reported a belief in big differences in negotiating styles of men and women—women were more cooperative, men more competitive. But this same research, replicated in the 1980s, failed to reproduce these conclusions. The researchers deduced that these earlier studies did not take power into account. When they considered the actions of those in positions of less power, including women, African-Americans, and others, women behaved in a manner similar to the others in corresponding positions. Here, as in Chapter Two, we observe the difficulty of disentangling the multiple contributing factors to perceived effectiveness. Race, gender, and power are three such factors.

The Costs and Benefits of Conflict in Health Care

Seeds of conflict in health care are ever present, given its mandate and profusion of strong and multiple professional cultures. Conflict is even more likely in the current environment of escalating stress produced by demands to spread too few resources over too many demands. What's at stake if such conflicts grow untended is significant. For the patient, the community, and the organization, it is health and the quality of life. Also affected are the institution's balance sheet and the perception of the organization or the profession in the community. What's at stake for the caregiver and health care leader are integrity, personal honor, and reputation. Additional costs are low morale and the impact of disputes on the quality of patient care, legal bills, lost staff time, and frazzled emotions (Marcus, 1995, p. 20).

Research from the Center for Creative Leadership in Greensboro, North Carolina, broadens our understanding of the costs of conflict in all organizations. "Insensitivity" to others was cited most commonly as the reason that executives and leaders in all industries fail (Cooper and Sawaf, 1997). Discord that goes untended is not just costly to executives who do not succeed—their organizations lose as well. According to the U.S. Department of Labor, 46 percent of those who quit their jobs in 1996 did so because they felt unappreciated. For those who remained, that perception was likely to be shared and lead to lower productivity, energy, and talent (Cooper and Sawaf, 1997, p. 50).

The benefits of conflict in organizations are no less important. GLHS contributors who offered their view of enduring leadership skills frequently cited the need for individuals to "play off" each other, to encourage conflict, and to seek and address variation among individuals who share a common purpose. As one contributor stated, "creativity is in the conflict. In fact, it's the source of creativity."

Peter Senge, highly regarded MIT professor of organization and management, states that teaching people how to *give up* being in agreement is key to unlocking openness at work: "We think agreement is so important. Who cares? You have to bring paradoxes, conflicts and dilemmas out in the open, so collectively we can be more intelligent than we can be individually" (Cooper and Sawaf, 1997, p. 103). Margaret Neale furthers this notion: "Groups are usually most concerned with managing or reducing conflict. Unfortunately, they are almost too good at this. They are conflict-averse, and in that aversion they lose the opportunity to raise different concerns and to be integrative."

Gender's Role in Health Care Leadership Conflicts

Health care's strong cultural traditions are not the only source of conflict in the field. Among others related to gender is a phenomenon known as validation or its lack. *Validation* is a gesture that acknowledges the importance of information and the granting of decision-making authority—and it is an important currency in health care. In meetings, for example, validation occurs when the leader acknowledges a participant's comment by saying, "That's an important point." Validation's opposite, invalidation, is signaled by gestures small and large, such as "ignoring a remark, negating a piece of information, or excluding a colleague's participation on the basis of prejudice, hierarchical standing, or interpersonal relations." Individuals are further invalidated when their conversational contributions are ignored, but later acknowledged when spoken by someone of higher status. Such invalidation is "common in gender, inter-professional and patient-provider relations" (Marcus and others, 1995, pp. 52–53).

As noted in Chapter One, at least a half-dozen female GLHS contributors volunteered their experiences with this phenomenon without knowing its name. One woman speaks for several: "Often in groups of men and women in meetings, I will say or suggest something, and no one takes it up. Four people later, 'Dave' or 'Tom' or 'Fred' offers the same idea and the people respond, 'That's a great idea!'"

This poses internal conflict for these women and leads to another personal struggle with perception: "Should I be more forceful? That is difficult, for I know I walk a fine line between being seen as 'forceful' and being seen as a 'bitch.'"

Invalidation and the attendant feelings it produces in women and men are distracting, thus detracting from whatever business is at hand (Marcus and others, 1995). The invalidators can become impatient by what the other person wants, and there is a "self-perception, often not hidden, of superiority. This can be seen in the ways men relate to women, doctors to nurses, administrators to clinicians, nurses to family members, and older people to younger people. This behavior reinforces the hierarchical nature of social ordering by demeaning the concerns and contributions of those considered less important" (pp. 52–53).

Proven Strategies for Working Well with Difference

The GLHS unearthed a variety of helpful methods for those who would better manage conflict while embracing its benefits. Although these can apply in any situation in which diversity is present, they are particularly useful when gender is the confounding aspect of the negotiation:

Negotiation Is Finding the Common Ground. Negotiation is a joint process of discovery occurring in stages and over time. The most effective tool for finding mutual interest is the good question, and the best way to enter a negotiation is with the intention of learning. Asking questions with an open mind can provide the answers. For example, health system executive and GLHS contributor Sharon Lee, R.N., M.B.A., uses this approach when she has difficulty with a physician: "If you have a problem with a colleague, you must ask yourself, what can we negotiate on?" Once common aims are clear, explicitly negotiate with those as the goal. Doing so refocuses the discussion on mutual interests rather than differences that are likely to remain.

Beware of Assumptions; Be Clear on Organizational Goals. Contributor Kathryn E. Johnson, president and CEO of the Healthcare Forum in San Francisco, notes that all negotiations are based on assumptions: "Through the process one should derive clarity of objectives and the mental models that are at play in the negotiation, while being sure that everyone is heard. This is best done through the inquiry/dialogue model. Through this process one can also identify the filters that are at the base of the positions people take."

Consider Your Own Biases. GLHS contributor Phyllis Kritek, coauthor of *Negotiating at an Uneven Table* (1994), encourages leaders who are negotiating to ask themselves how they contribute to their own conflicts: "Males and females are a bundle of different opinions—no matter how decisive we appear to others. All conflict is 'relational'— then in healthcare we add the elements of high stakes, unclear 'rules' of the game, the changing nature of the game . . . and different interpretations of information and its meaning." Being clear about our own biases is essential for negotiating well.

Think Systemically. Many health care decisions are intricately related with others, often at different scales of intensity and importance. GLHS contributor Cathy Michaels, Ph.D., R.N., believes that health care decisions are multidimensional—affecting the individual involved as well as family members, and then larger groups beyond. She suggests imagining a matrix showing those who will be affected by the decision. She acknowledges that doing this is difficult, but in her own community nursing practice she successfully moves consensus-based recommendations from individuals to the group and larger community.

Quick Closure Is Not Always Best. We need to become more comfortable with waiting; at times, greater consideration will produce a more innovative path. Contributor Donna Fosbinder, D.N.S., R.N., notes that "self-renewal and reflection pay off here—both these help in not getting lost in 'reaction'."

Use Language to Reframe the Issues. Stating concerns in the context of mutual interests is important to successful negotiations and decisions, as we have seen. Just the simple exchange of the word "and" for "but" can be a powerful and transforming act leading to more productive conversation. This signals the search for interests that are complementary rather than competitive.

Construct Groups for Maximum Generativity. Health care leaders create and interact with groups of colleagues many times weekly. Some form through natural selection, in which the common base of membership is similarity, proximity, or prior acquaintance. These groups have strong potential for smooth relationships but minimal potential for problem solving and learning, for they lack the diversity required for the tasks. Creating groups of individuals with natural affinity but who possess unique kinds of information may be most effective for creativity (Gruenfeld, Mannix, Williams, and Neale, 1996).

Honor Emotion, Pay Attention, and Be Open to Inner Wisdom. Mohandas (Mahatma) Ghandi believed that responsibility involved our wholehearted willingness to pay attention. This advice applies to honoring ourselves as well as the situations around us. Among other benefits, this practice provides us access to intuition. The inner wisdom of intuition is an important resource for creativity and conflict resolution at the highest levels of leadership. Persuasive research shows that the most effective decision making is not reached through calls to eliminate emotion and passion from management: eighty-two of the ninety-three winners of the Nobel Prize over sixteen years believe that intuition plays an important role in creative and scientific discoveries (Cooper and Sawaf, 1997, p. 63).

Be Aware of Producing an Adversarial Situation. GLHS contributor Neale believes that many people perceive the situations they are in to be adversarial, even if they are not necessarily that way. Why? They do not know how to do otherwise, says Neale, and, therefore, "The negotiations *will be* adversarial. They will obfuscate the issues, keep their cards close to their chests, play power games; make efforts to keep their opponents off balance—and generally 'mess with their opponents' minds.'" If the goal is mutually rewarding relationships with the parties, the better route is to identify issues of shared concern, she advises.

The Changing Paradigm of Power

At its most simple level, power is currency. Power at this level is gender neutral. For Roxane Spitzer and other GLHS contributors, power in health care is simply the ability to get things done—and this is a critical element of the leader's job.

Yet our leadership experiences with power when combined with gender are not usually so simple. Spitzer, for example, suggests that when men and women show their power, it has decidedly different effects on their audiences. Men may receive confirmation and support for their actions. In contrast, women who take action may actually lose power, especially if they have female staff, she says. Neither of these assertions is surprising in light of the male-oriented models of leadership as well as females' frequent wishes for symmetry when working with one another.

Another commonly accepted view of power is the use of authority, control, and influence over others. It is useful to consider author and anthropologist Riane Eisler's view (1987, p. 193) as another way of describing the stereotypical male form of leadership. For Eisler, power is often synonymous with domination *over* other people rather than power achieved through working *with* other people.

How then do we identify the factors that make for successful use of power for both women and men? Although it is difficult to identify true cause-and-effect relationships between power and gender, the experiences of GLHS contributors are instructive. Their approaches offer diverse points of view.

Jennifer Kozakowski, R.N., M.H.A., a successful senior executive with a managed care firm in Los Angeles, sees a split between what she calls "synergic" power and "egoic" power. "Egoic power is 'win/lose' power—power in which the players are really playing hard ball," she says. "But with synergic power, my gain is your gain. Exercising egoic power means you've got to go to war, it means you crawl over anybody, anything to get what you want. While there is a time and place for this, one must understand the consequences of pursuing this in health care. . . . Health care is quite village-like, even though it is a big business. Anybody could be your next boss. Also, people are afraid of brutal people. Yes, you get results, you get work from people—you get enough. But you don't get the cream."

A female consultant to senior executives sees an ongoing cultural trajectory in health care in which power is being amassed in the few and the numbers of the disempowered are growing. She warns, "Definition, allocation, and use of power are at the nexus of the future of health care organizations—and the scramble to survive. And, health care is definitely a survival-driven industry. People perceive the need to amass power."

A male GLHS contributor and national figure in health care distinguishes between power, influence, and authority: "Power is positional—e.g., I have the gun—I have the power. You have the gun—you have the power. Influence is more lasting; it transitions situations. Power is a double-edged sword. It's important to know when to transition from power to influence. I very seldom use true power or authority."

Cathy Michaels sees power as accountability: "Most people try to give their own power away to a leader or to a cause. Yet to keep it is to take a risk and to be vulnerable. To give it away is to be less than our full selves."

When considering the relationship of power, domination, and dysfunction, Carol Pearson, author of *The Hero Within*, is helpful: "The outsider almost always comes to understand that those in power consciously or unconsciously rig the contest. Affirmative action [for example] as typically practiced, means that women and minorities, to be seen as worthy, are expected to live up to a pattern designed by white men in their own image" (Pearson, 1989, p. 93).

Although the GLHS did not focus exclusively on power, the subject still brought forth emotionally charged feeling and beliefs from many contributors. Their comments and concerns are summarized here:

- The difference in working with those who share power with others, compared with those who exercise power unilaterally, is tremendous. When the latter model is used frequently, it is off-putting and counterproductive. The result worsens when variables such as differences in clinical training (doctors and nurses, clinicians, and others) come into play.

- For some, winning isn't the same as it used to be. Kozakowski says, "Some men still play these games, and some women who reach these [high] levels play them, too. Perhaps that's because they've been put upon for

so long, now they're the ones to put it on someone else.
Now some men are moving away from egoic power, and
they are trying to learn the good skills that women
have had."

• Many GLHS contributors believe that power is tran-
sient. Several espouse a "use *and* lose" attitude toward
power rather than the more traditional, egoic model of
power they still see—the "use *or* lose" approach.

Power as Influence Without Manipulation

The foundation and focus of management in the last two hundred
years has been external power, analysis, and technical rationality,
often overshadowing qualities such as spirit, emotion, wisdom, and
intuition. But today a new kind of emotional intelligence is being
acknowledged, and it is at work everywhere in business culture,
including health care.

This emotional intelligence produces influence without manip-
ulation or authority. Key to the emerging model of leadership and
management is the recognition that the role of power has changed—
power is now encompassing "perceiving, learning, relating, inno-
vating . . . and acting in ways that take into account emotional
valence." The traditional ways of competing are being replaced by
opportunities to influence and to operate in two realities simultaneously, one of both conflict and cooperation, chaos and collaboration. These are called *business ecosystems* (Cooper and Sawaf,
1997, pp. 181–182).

A clear distinction can be made between the power of position
and effective leadership. Study participant Hudson Birden, M.P.H.,
health officer for New Britain, Connecticut, believes "being a manager, a boss, provides one *positional* power. To be a true leader, however, one must engender respect and trust . . . one must do this
without having to depend on the superficial qualities and trappings

of position. You can use them all, and still get things done through bullying, etc., but you don't get real buy-in or allegiance where you don't have to ask—other people *want* to come along."

One GLHS contributor, a successful female CEO of several hospitals, believes power comes from guiding. She says she spends a lot of time teaching and telling stories to all stakeholders, framing the same message differently for various audiences. She feels teaching is an essential part of leadership because some groups, including boards, lack understanding of the issues because they're not close enough to health care every day. She believes that women are more oriented than men toward communicating and teaching, and spells out her approach to communication: "I integrate humor, I integrate different types of information to build richness; I engage others and I have a certain amount of charisma."

Women, Success in Leadership Roles, and Power

Recalling that Tannen and others propose that symmetry is important in women's relationships, it is understandable that the old paradigm of power—power over, rather than power with—brings forth uncomfortable feelings in many women. In the face of power expressed traditionally—some win while others lose—having such power is frequently perceived by women as selfish.

Women receive mixed messages about power and competition, often stimulating profound feelings of ambivalence about not simply holding power but also being competitive and exhibiting success and prosperity. In an exercise developed for the Center for Nursing Leadership by JoEllen Koerner, Ph.D., R.N., participants focused on women, success, and prosperity. The premise was that this is a new age for women and that it is natural for them to be powerful and to prosper. The definition of prosperity was to experience a balanced life, including the mental, physical, emotional, spiritual, and financial levels. Participants in the exercise shared their feelings about prosperity, and many expressed some unease about having it. As noted in Koerner's exercise: "Women have associated being successful in the world with being male. As we cross an invisible role line and learn to become stronger, more independent, we feel an uneasiness that tells us we are approaching some [contrary] earlier programming" (Koerner, 1996).

As we have seen, reasons for female ambivalence are clearer when we consider how power has been displayed. Borysenko, too, reminds us (1996) that many women may fear taking leadership roles because of their awareness of how power has been amassed and abused through the millennia.

Study contributor Katherine W. Vestal, Ph.D., R.N., believes that for females in health care, using power "is an art, for which we do not get enough training. We take 'it' personally and internalize events around us. People can be powerful and not be ruthless. Most leaders don't realize their own power." Kathryn E. Johnson agrees that women personalize issues, also observing that they don't get over losses gracefully: "When competition really heats up, women will back off. It is more difficult for them, they are more modest in their statements of accomplishment, and they may be less interested in 'winning' for their own personal achievement."

Stepping Forward With Power

When women overcome their ambivalence about garnering and using their power in ways that facilitate the work of others rather than constrict them, they help themselves while also creating renewed organizations. Roxane Spitzer is instructive on gender and power and their relationship to the qualities of such organizations: "In organizations where the effective use of power is viewed as sharing power, the female style of being people-oriented, expressing a desire to share resources, and building interdependent relationships reflects the traditional way women have been socialized to use power in this country. Women have learned in their roles as wives and mothers to serve as a resource and a source of support to those around them, a skill transferred by many women to the workplace. Women have also learned that by facilitating success for others they are respected and consulted. Often the mere act of empowerment increases one's personal power, a critical concept in today's transformed healthcare organizations" (Spitzer, 1997, p. 732).

According to the findings of Aburdene and Naisbitt (1992), women glean their power from their internal spirit and inner strength rather than from external sources. GLHS contributor Gates McKibbin, Ph.D., strategy consultant to organizations inside and outside health care, offers positive steps for women to take to resolve their ambivalence and move ahead with freedom and excellence in their executive practices. Reflecting Aburdene and Naisbitt's message, McKibbin defines power as coming from a person's deepest sense of soul and spirit. Women, she continues, must do "our inner work so we can be as powerful as we're capable of—it's denied and thwarted so much. The only way we're going to have the healing is if we do our own work first. Based on that, we need to support each other in authenticity and not in our illusion of strength."

Other GLHS participants offered options, perspectives, and approaches to developing comfort and facility with power:

Become Bilingual; Use Power With and Power Over. During the study, there were clear calls for both women and men to become comfortable using *all* the tools available for effective leadership— not just those that gender and culture make familiar. Certain skills, such as exercising the authority of position, are still best when quick action is called for. These skills and attitudes may never become second nature for some women, but they can and should be developed and used.

Speak Clearly and Concisely. Being assertive is one way women and men alike can express power. Verbally, assertive behavior balances being polite with being direct. Most girls learn an indirect, "polite" communications style, whereas most men issue commands and criticisms with no added language intended to make others feel comfortable with the message. For example, women use less demanding language and frequently couch their statements with "Okay?" or "Is that all right?" to soften their impact. Men's statements are usually more direct, clear, and brief. Theirs is the language of the powerful who need not fear giving offense.

Beware of Unconscious Passive Behavior. Nonverbal cues also indicate assertiveness, or its lack, in both men and women. With passive behavior, for example, eye contact is often poor, posture may be slumped, and a whining tone may accompany the message. Assertive behavior includes direct eye contact, the speaker standing or sitting tall, and a firm, moderate voice intonation. Other messages conveying power are such small gestures as the space we occupy in meetings. Contributor Kathy Reno, R.N., M.B.A., says women must consider where they sit in a meeting—literally: "Women don't usually sit at the head of the table. We will usually try to convey 'community.' But do we give away power when we do that?"

Notice the Effect of Your Growing Power on the Women Around You. Women are often concerned with how they display power around men—they have experienced other women who are considered ballsy, a bitch, or worse. But there's another consideration as well: "When we choose a direct style with another woman, we need to consider how . . . other women might personalize our confrontation and react emotionally. We can take the time in these situations to assure we have communicated our point effectively and to leave the other person with a positive sense of her worth" (Duff, 1993, p. 199). A woman may take solace in knowing that as she evolves with authenticity, incorporating new personal power, she will eventually reap respect and trust among her colleagues. Patience may be required as others who are still ambivalent about power catch up with the true integrity of your new leadership practice.

Use Power Like Currency. GLHS contributor David Kindig urges women to "get comfortable with what power is, what you have, and how you exert it. Realize it's an asset to be gathered and spent, as part of your fiduciary responsibility." Contributor Sister Mary Jean

Ryan, president of SSM Health System, encourages women to "get comfortable with power. I have it, and I like having it. I can get things done with it. I consider abuse of power to be not just its overuse, but its underuse as well. We [women] are not good at using it for good things as well as we might."

Embrace Your Maturity. Women in their twenties and thirties who are emerging as leaders are encouraged to bring forward their fresh perspectives while also honing their skills and developing themselves. Women beyond these ages are more seasoned professionals, and they experience the changing nature of power for a woman as she ages. I have seen repeatedly in my own colleagues and the many women in the GLHS the evolution of power in women as they reach beyond their early mothering years. As we shall see in Chapter Nine, these women are vigorous and they have reaped the benefits of maturation as professionals as well as the seasoning that family responsibilities often brings. They are in "possession of a kind of fierce power that is biologically mediated, yet there is no fear that these women will become a cadre of fierce, masculine warriors . . . it is not warranted by female physiology" (Borysenko, 1996, p. 7).

Hone Your Instincts for Power and Timing. GLHS contributor Alma Koch believes women either "have a nose for power, or they develop it with experience. It is important [to do this], but not critical in one's early years." People who understand power have an innate sense of timing. They are able to put an issue on the table, pull back, and look at who the players are. She adds, "You have to become an opportunist and you must understand the bigger environment."

Focus on Competence and Skill. Koch continues, "In health care, one can achieve based on competence and experience. Power is not as important in industries that are not competency-based—this is one of the reasons that women are not as motivated by power, but achievement." Another contributor described her close colleague as a model of such proficiency. A female physician of great national regard whose time commitments precluded her from participating in the study, she is effective because she has extraordinarily good analytic skills. Yet she has also gone beyond them. According to the study contributor who works closely with her, "She stays on a conceptual level and doesn't get distracted by the details or the politics. Quickly, she considers a situation and she educates her colleagues to see new factors. She is willing to change her mind and she can isolate distracting phenomena such as politics or where the money flow is. She also speaks very well, is decisive, and very good at stating and defending her positions."

Recognize What Is and Isn't in Your Control. Contributor Robert Boyle is an accomplished health care executive in acute care and medical group practice settings. "Wisdom and power lay in recognizing the factors that are not in your control," he says. "One can be a perfect leader, and it still may not work out."

Recognize that Old Behaviors May No Longer Be Necessary. Some women best serve themselves by developing additional leadership skills such as direct communication and comfort with power, but others do well to scale back undue exercise of these same behaviors. Several GLHS contributors cited usually older females whom they consider to be aggressive, not assertive. One contributor's view speaks for several: "I have noticed that women who are in the committees [in my national policy organization] are uncommonly aggressive—even though they do not need to be any longer. But they have needed to be that way before."

Access the Points of Highest Leverage. GLHS contributor Barbara Donaho, R.N., M.S., is one of the most successful nurse executives in the history of U.S. health care, amassing a series of firsts for women and for nurses as she has progressed through elected positions of influence in national organizations, including the American Hospital Association. "For me," she says, "power means understanding the leverage point and how to make the broadest impact." Donaho's choices of national leadership roles reflect careful focus on high-impact opportunities that match her leadership priorities for the field.

Avoid Self-Serving Leadership. Looking out for Number One will probably pay off only in the short term. Donaho says, "If you are self-serving, you will not last. Once you are seen that way, you will lose opportunities and will not be sought out."

Cherish Mistakes. Today's management literature often reveres making mistakes. But little of it offers examples, particularly for women, of how less-than-positive results can be turned into opportunities for greater power and influence. GLHS participant Navy Captain (retired) Jane Swanson, R.N., gives an example. In her twenty-six-year career with the Navy, Swanson seldom had direct line authority. Still, she rose to head a national organization of four hundred thousand nurses and was elevated to the top 1 percent of nurses in her branch of the service. "My leadership career," she says, "has been a gradual process in which I have learned not just how to listen, but how to *hear* without putting up internal walls." Four or five years ago she developed an empowerment program, which, she says, she "essentially crammed down the throats" of her colleagues. This went on for three cycles until she observed that her intentions weren't being realized. "I made a mistake," she says, "and I admitted I made a mistake. That gave me considerable credibility, and the level of dialogue among us was lifted."

Stop Competing and Manage Upward. Contributor Heidi Boerstler notes that one way to power is to "always make your boss and team look good. Talk them up. Then they will fight for you. Get over the competing stuff and think they are terrific!" Contributor Wanda Jones observes that many women do not know how to manage upward. They work hard, she says, to manage across their peer groups and their subordinates, but they don't do much about managing their senior teams—for example, by telling "the story" to the board. Why not? Often, she says, women are "waiting to be asked."

Develop Personal Power. Contributor Nancy Valentine, Ph.D., R.N., occupies one of the most powerful positions in world health care as the U.S. Veterans Administration's senior nurse. She observes:

"Personal power is more important than positional power. Key ingredients for personal power are effective communication, the ability to read situations, move situations forward, try out ideas, push the 'envelope' [take risks] and stay grounded."

Summing Up

This chapter covers background and success strategies for the first of the important antidotes to personal, cultural, and professional challenges to women who strive for excellence in their leadership practice. Negotiation, conflict, and power are of a piece. Taken together and practiced with skill, they enhance any leader's perceived competence, effectiveness, and personal and collegial respect. Chapter Six offers an in-depth perspective of the next key leadership skill: communicating for maximum effectiveness.

6

Antidote 2: Using Communication as a Bridge

Despite thirty-five years of recognition for his abilities as a leader, William Gonzalez feels there is one skill so complex and so important that he will never completely master it. Gonzalez, president and CEO of the Butterworth Health System in Grand Rapids, Michigan, believes he is "never good enough" when it comes to honing his talent for communication.

This chapter focuses on ways to enhance this all-powerful tool by examining the following:

- Key socialization and communication differences between men and women on the job, and how these come forward in health care

- Perceptions of female leaders whose communication styles do not match those that are associated with clear and decisive leadership

- How women can be recognized as competent when the "male" model of leadership is at play

- Options and skills for effective presentation

Exploring Communication Differences

Differences in communication style and meaning have profound implications for our workplace interactions, particularly if they are not acknowledged or understood. Conversation has a ritualistic nature, and when everyone involved understands "the rules," communication can flow smoothly. But often people don't understand each other's rules and preferences. For example: Is averting one's eyes evasive or polite? Is meeting another's gaze engaging or aggressive? Is waiting for another to finish speaking respectful or hesitant? Is seeking the opinions of others inclusive or indecisive?

To understand the full measure of communication rituals, answer these questions from your own perspective first. Then answer them as a coworker would, preferably one who is not a friend. Are your answers different? Undoubtedly some are—and here we begin to appreciate both the richness and challenge of effective communication.

Communication is said to be the soul of management, and clear messages influence people to act. Communication, then, is a key aspect of power, as we saw in Chapter Five. Strong communication skills are required by health care leaders for a host of reasons, ranging from personal interactions when caring for patients and their families to inspiring others within the team, organization, and larger community. Focusing on the latter roles, health care leaders must be able to call on strong communications skills to do the following (Robinson, 1993):

- Motivate, captivate, and persuade audiences in multiple groups and communities inside and outside the organization

- Prevent, contain, manage, and resolve crises

- Enhance understanding and collaboration among diverse employee and community groups

- Coordinate and nurture excellence within the team, organization, or department

- Inspire leadership in others

- Improve decision making among health care professional care teams and other leaders

A successful nurse executive who contributed to the GLHS considered her communication tasks in light of gender. She asked two male physician colleagues, "How can I be heard more effectively?" The first, a department head, responded: "I'm not sure you ever could." "Why?" she asked. He replied, "Because physicians are paranoid about the future. They have huge resentments." The second physician added: "You are a woman, and a guy always filters gender in his thinking." The nurse executive was "absolutely shocked." She believes that this trait is one of males, not physicians, because they do the "gender thing" by taking into consideration first whether a man or a woman is speaking. "I do not imagine that women do the same thing," she says. "Part of this filtering by men determines how they decide the merit of what the person is going to say." How can women deal with this? She says, "There is absolutely nothing you can do—except be consistent and don't worry. But this adds up to a real problem. I really didn't think that gender issues were quite that deep."

Socialization Differences at Work

By now it is well established that there are custom, language, and dialect differences between the sexes. As Tannen (1990) asserts, for example: "For men, conversations are often negotiations in which people try to achieve and to maintain the upper hand." As we have seen previously, women often use conversation for connection and as a negotiation for confirmation and support.

In an analysis of men's and women's networks, Dalinger found that males generally communicate to fulfill a task function and females normally communicate to fulfill the social-emotional function. Building on the social-emotional theme, linguist Robin Lakoff found that women need to be in constant communication in order to preserve feelings of trust (Duff, 1993, p. 197). This is important for women, for much of their perceived success and fulfillment at work is based on trust. Women who don't conform to these "rules of talk" can be viewed with suspicion by other women.

Anthropologist Marjorie Harness Goodwin found that girls criticize other girls who call attention to their own attributes or performance, saying things like "she thinks she's so cute," or similar comments. She concludes that talking in ways that display self-confidence is simply not approved for girls. She and other anthropologists found that girls get better results with other girls if they phrase their ideas as suggestions rather than orders, and if they give reasons for their suggestions that include the group's well-being (Tannen, 1994, p. 36). This indirect style of communicating has distressing consequences in real leadership instances later in life—in a word, the female leader communicating in this manner may be viewed as less competent than her male counterparts. Later in this chapter we see evidence of this dynamic, as well as ways to mitigate it, in health care management contexts.

Gender Communication Differences at Work

Several authors and GLHS contributors commented on the ways gender differences affect leadership and patient care transactions.

Female Physician's Communicating Style Builds Relationships. A high percentage of patients report that they are dissatisfied with the ways their physicians communicate with them. Noted economist Eli Ginzberg suggests that the fact that many women communicate more with their patients can be viewed as a gain in terms of patient satisfaction, as we saw in Chapter One. He speculates that there are long-term economic benefits to this behavior, even after the higher costs of these visits are fully considered (Friedman, 1994, pp. 140–141).

Looking Below the Surface. Perhaps these interactions occur because a female physician wants to know more about the "whole" patient—to the end of gaining a deeper understanding of the dimensions of the patient's complaint and course of treatment. Wanda Jones describes this same phenomenon in the administrative suite: "Men are more inclined to buy the package, and the position. Women 'look under the suit' and see the personal side, and are thus able to see more of the truth and more about key relationships."

Being Subtle. In her thirty years working as a health care spokeswoman and consultant in many hospitals, GLHS interviewee Jones has seen distinctive male and female communication patterns: in her view, men often dominate discussions and sometimes make dogmatic, unsupported statements, whereas women wait to speak. When they do speak, they usually just confirm what someone else has said, suggest process steps, or communicate facts without an opinion. She says, "The women often come up to me in the hall afterwards to offer important background that is too politically sensitive to be mentioned in meetings. It seems to be taken for granted that women are expected to tolerate and sometimes overlook immature behavior of the men while remaining calm and accepting."

"Puffing" and Other Signals. Body language also contains gender-coded messages. One female GLHS contributor who is a consultant based in the midwest has frequently observed male body language in board rooms. She believes that these messages are based on the premise that "the more space you occupy, the more power you have." She observes, "The male body position is one leg is up, ankle across the other knee forming an 'A,' with hands behind the head. Or, they will put one arm across the next guy's chair." She calls this behavior "puffing." She recounted a recent meeting with a hospital CEO to whom she was reporting that the nurses felt leadership is "in their way." She says, "The CEO began puffing all over—putting his hands behind his head, even putting both his legs on top of the board room table."

She continues: "Female body language is usually quite different. Women are taught not to cross their legs in this manner, to fold their arms, and to assume smaller spaces. This sends a message that this meeting or this space is 'not about me, it's about you.'" Donna Wright, R.N., M.S., a GLHS contributor and consultant to nurses nationally, provides important perspective. Wright observes that words don't mean much—"they are only 7 percent of the message. This type of body position equals the statement 'It's okay to push me over.'" Wright uses role playing to show how female nurses communicate with one another, and often observes women trying to tend to the other's needs. "Each often demonstrates body language that is tight and low, and then the other starts to drop even lower," she says. These behaviors are often unconscious, so Wright suggests videotaping as a way of to receive helpful feedback. She also advises that nurses and other female leaders consider the puffing option themselves, particularly in abusive situations.

Another way for women to equalize the communication flow when talking to men is to assess each situation on its own merits. One contributor, who describes herself as a big woman and comfortable with her size, says she has learned to sit down when dealing with men who are smaller than she. Men, she says, never have to think about how they are perceived—they want to be, or assume they are, in the power position. Dealing with them on an equal footing, so to speak, has been aided by this relatively simple adjustment in body posture.

Is Anyone Listening? One contributor described his experience with the management team—all men except for the vice president of nursing—that he inherited some years ago when he became president and CEO. "When I came, the VP of nursing let me know she didn't feel she was being treated very well," he says. "I noticed that at meetings, she couldn't get a word in and that she was on the 'meek side'—once she tried to say something, she wouldn't try again." How did he handle this? "I had to resort to a kindergarten-like state. In the meetings, I would go back and ask her what she had wanted to say, or I had to interrupt others when she wanted to speak. I had to do this for months—and the guys just didn't get it. Eventually she started raising her hand."

Perceptions of Competence in Women Leaders

Vincent Covello, president of Covello Communications, a New York-based communications consultant and former professor of public health at Columbia University, is an expert in advising leaders who communicate in situations of high concern and low trust.

Sought out by senior U.S. government officials and leaders in many industries, he is particularly well known in public health practice for his advice on handling communication about conditions of great public concern.

Covello has conducted extensive research that reviewed situations in which people are worried, upset, or angry about what's happened or what might happen. "High concern," a term that implies low trust, is a statement of concern about matters of health—the quality of life, costs incurred, or other economic and aesthetic issues.

A perceived loss or potential threat to something of value—health and safety issues, goals within a department, or employment security, to name a few disparate examples–prompts high concern. According to Covello, people form initial perceptions of trust and credibility within thirty to sixty seconds of meeting someone, and these perceptions are very resistant to change. In fact, they can be the filters through which all further information is passed. Covello's fifteen years of research have revealed three components of trust: the perception of caring, the perception of competence, and the perception of honesty and openness. He bases his conclusions on the supposition that perception equals reality.

Daily interactions for most health care executives are mixed with situations of low concern and high concern. Covello's work has important implications for female leaders. Usually, concern is low in routine events such as regularly scheduled department meetings. Health care experts and support personnel regularly come together in these settings, and the primary determinant of trust in these everyday instances is competence. Women and men therefore are most successful when they are well prepared and present themselves confidently.

But in situations of high concern, much more weight is given to caring and empathy. Covello's research shows that women have higher ratings on these qualities, reflecting the stereotypes we explored earlier: that females are more empathetic and open. But he has also found that females are seen as less competent than males.

There *is* good news for women in this. First, they are perceived to be more credible in high-concern situations because of their caring and honesty. Second, a clear path exists to mitigate the problem of perceived lack of competency. Covello's findings indicate that people are willing to accept compensatory evidence, but in situations of high concern they focus more on the negative. Therefore, the presenter needs three times more qualitative or quantitative evidence to overcome that negative perception. So the goal in high-concern situations is to provide facts and to generate trust and credibility. Although perception equals reality, his studies also report that individual credibility always overrides group perception.

But unfortunately the news for women isn't all good. Regardless of how successful a woman is in communicating competence in high-concern situations—in other words, in displaying caring, competency, and honesty—the male is still accorded more credibility! Because a man starts behind a woman in trust and credibility, if he provides evidence of his caring and empathy along with his competence, he ends up farther ahead.

Unfortunately, Covello's research even in the late 1990s shows little or no change in perceptions for most groups, except for those younger than thirty-five. For them, there is more refusal to accept stereotypes.

Covello's research and experiences in low-trust high-concern situations are comparable to those encountered by female leaders in health care who still face the dominant male leadership model. They serve as the foundation for the tips in the following list.

Ways to Create the Perception of Competency

- Simply be competent—skillful, knowledgeable, and clear about the issue at hand. This is by far the best antidote to group perceptions of competence in concern-causing situations.

- When it is called for, indicate a mastery of fact and detail. Covello believes that often women must demonstrate knowledge at an encyclopedic level. According to him, the best example of this is found in the film *My Cousin Vinnie*, in which the Marisa Tomei character gave excruciatingly detailed facts about an overhead cam engine—testimony that proved a defendant's innocence.

- Be organized, disciplined, and methodical. In the workplace, according to Covello, being messy implies a lack of expertise, which is a subindicator of competence.

- Don't rely on prepared notes or read a speech. Covello says, "This is one of the worst things a woman can do—it shows you are dependent upon your notes. Maybe you didn't even write them! People are thinking, 'If you are an expert, why do you have to read it?'"

- Pay attention to subtle cues, such as blinking at normal rates and keeping your hands open and at waist level.

- Carefully use endorsements. Noting awards, degrees, and achievements are important indicators of competence. Although women are wise to use these in presentations, they must do so without "tooting their horns."

- Take care with language asking for consensus and vocal characteristics such as breaks in the voice, high pitch, and too many "uhs" and "ahs." Use language that is authoritative, definitive, well organized, and embodied in short sentences. Examples of tentative and less-commanding language are "maybe," "probably," "let's," "depending," and "try to." Use "will" or "will not" instead.

- Never say "I'm not an expert"—instead, tell them what you are. In situations of high concern about leadership's intentions or competence, such a disclaimer can add to already existing confusion. When people are confused about the message, they will blame the messenger.

Assessing These Lessons for Female Health Care Leaders

We have much to learn as we move from the dominant leadership mode of "one right way" to the new mode of accepting multiple contributions to a better way. Adopting wholesale the lessons of communicating in the dominant mode and discrediting yet again more traditionally feminine ways of speaking, acting, and doing would be an unfortunate step backward. Women walk a slippery slope—Should they adapt their communication styles to the dominant culture? Or should they speak their own language, helping to create a culture that embraces multiple ways of bringing forth results?

They may do both. Women and men alike may be dedicated to the goal of increased cultural respect with regard to gender and race, yet they may still consciously choose the dominant communication style to accomplish a certain task. The important thing is to choose consciously, aligning the best style with the goal to be achieved.

Communicating for Effectiveness: Strengthening Women's Voices

As central as assertiveness is to being powerful as a leader, so too is it key to communicating effectively. This can be challenging for women, as we have seen, for many have been raised to believe that being direct and assertive invites being perceived as hard, bitchy, or worse. It's challenging for men too, for they have been brought up in the same social system.

Interviewee Pam Thompson, R.N., offered her view of the struggle of assertiveness versus aggressiveness. "I've never heard a man called shrill," she says. "Aggressive men get things done. Aggressive women get stamped on. I don't say this much, but this isn't fair." She is teaching her teenage daughter to be assertive, a word she didn't learn until she was nineteen or twenty. Pam recalls the all-too-familiar dynamic of invalidation discussed in Chapter Five—she suggests an idea to a group that isn't recognized until one of the men says the same thing fifteen minutes later. This irks her, but she sees it as a process dilemma. "It is helpful to detach and know that's the process of the group," she says. "It's not just one or the same person taking my ideas, and it's within the same group of people. If I brought this up, they would deny they are doing it."

GLHS contributor Sister Mary Jean Ryan approaches this situation with a different focus. She says, "Women should speak up, literally. They should speak in a louder voice." She continues, "Say something in a meeting early on, too. I notice that if I wait, I won't speak. It's almost as if I'm waiting for a hole in the conversation." A hospital system CEO, Sister Ryan was invited to a meeting convened by the governor of Missouri at which she was the only woman. During the meeting, she asked a question and made several comments. She speculates on why one of the group later commended her for being selected: "Was I given credibility because of the number of questions I asked, or was it the substance of the comments?"

Contributor Judy Miller, R.N., has also learned how to speak up and speak directly and clearly: "Once I got into the executive suite, I did not speak the language, I wasn't always clear, and I was often not listened to." Among other things Miller has learned, "Men listen to other men and I think they agree because of the tone of voice."

Communication experts agree with these highly successful female leaders. GLHS interviewee Joan Kenley, Ph.D., is an expert in voice communication, but she is not just any expert. Her voice is that of the ubiquitous digitized operator of directory assistance in almost all U.S. cities. She is also a clinical psychologist, voice coach, and author of *Voice Power: A Breakthrough Method to Enhance Your Speaking Voice* (1988). Her work offers important insights into the vocal stereotypes at play in our professional interactions. Several studies of spoken English reveal, for example, that low-pitched, clear voices are judged to be more mature and truthful, whereas high-pitched, nasal voices signal low status. And standards for women and men are different—both sexes prefer male voices that are clear and deep, and female voices that have a certain amount of "breathiness" to them. Unfortunately, however, many people associate breathiness with passivity and low-pitched voice clarity with power (Franklin, 1995, pp. 38, 41).

Kenley's voice tips for women:

- Use of the voice is mostly learned, for the voice is a socially trained instrument. Relax and open up your voice so that you always have available that voice that communicates exactly what you want it to.

- If you want a "head tone," you can go up there; if you want a "gut tone," you can go down there.

- Women often assume "sliding and melodic" voices with men, which are a more emotional form of communication that *captivates* rather than *activates* men. Clearly state and prove your case and select the vocal tones that match the messages so men can hear them appropriately.

Context and Purpose as Final Arbiters

Context and purpose are always key to selecting a communication style. GLHS contributor Wanda Jones describes instances in which indirect communication is clearly not effective. For example, instead of making clear proposals at meetings or in writing, women "hint" and then talk about their ideas in the halls. "No one has to listen to a hint," says Jones, who points out that most male executives are trained to act on something proposed in writing. The impact of doing this is that the proposal is talked over with several people and may be presented in committees. "This is being clear, and is taking responsibility for one's ideas," she points out. "This would lead to untold power if women were to do this."

Expanding communication skills permits choice about how much visibility, directness, and credibility are needed. Now head of the San Francisco Foundation and recently the head of the San Francisco Department of Health, physician Sandra Hernandez says she "gets the biggest kick" out of working behind the scene and likes making others look good. She also enjoys people calling for opinion even if she's not part of the official decision-making team. Working from behind, as she calls it, allows her to kill bad ideas, identify potentially problematic areas, and create programs that are very well received, such as a drug treatment "on demand" program, which she and others instituted in San Francisco in the late 1990s. "Everyone is claiming success for the program, from the Mayor to the Board of Supervisors," she says. "This pleases me greatly, and is an example of exerting power by influence rather than authority."

Hernandez's generosity is an example of discernment in a woman who recognizes the efforts of others as well as honoring her own accomplishments. Having established herself as a leader, she can afford to step back from the limelight and allow others to claim success. In doing so, she is effective as team member, mentor, and influencer. However, this kind of leadership is not always possible for women who are still establishing themselves. Clearly, there are times when it is appropriate to reveal accomplishments and step forward rather than back.

Discernment is also key to communicating well in heated conversations. When joining such a conversation, do so with a deliberately slow speech pattern, which allows discord to continue, say Cooper and Sawaf (1997). This disarms the discord and "engages the creative energies of the group without permitting any of the individuals to attack one another." They also suggest that making feelings and thoughts "visible" by using phrases such as "here's what I think, and here's how I got there; I assumed that, and I came to this conclusion because" can balance advocacy with inquiry.

Presentation and Effective Communication

Rena Spence is a successful health care executive who speaks to the importance of personal stature, believing that the route to power for women is not very different from that for men. She counsels that success depends largely on the "presentation of self": "Barring external impediments, those people who achieve leadership positions have a set of internal qualities that persuade others to trust an organization to their hands."

Corroborating the concern about self-esteem discussed in Chapter Four, Spence identifies these qualities as "confidence in oneself, a willingness to take risks; perseverance; and most important, the ability to not take personally the negative consequences of organizational decision making. It is not the technical qualifications that hinder women in leadership positions, but rather that women have yet to develop the self-confidence or the sense of presentation that is essential in these roles" (Friedman, 1994, p. 246).

As women assume roles of greater leadership responsibility, they confront more aspects of the male model of leadership. One of these is physical presentation—the expectation of a crisp, professional look and affect that still signify corporate stewardship. Except for the white coats and scrubs of clinicians and other scientists, corporate dress is the norm in most health care settings.

GLHS contributor Jane Neubauer says she knows that appearance is just marketing and superficial nonsense, but that it still works. She recounts an experience about twelve years ago during her first week as a CEO: "I entered a room of twenty men with bald heads, red ties, and gray suits. I was in my silk turquoise suit. I felt so conspicuous, and several people got up to get me a seat." Since then, she has been more careful about what she wears depending on where she is going. "I want them to hear what I say rather than focus on how I look, at least until I get to know them a bit," she adds.

GLHS contributor Mary Richardson, Ph.D., said she read John Molloy's *Dress for Success* some years ago, and knew "inside" that his advice that women look "like men"—dress in gray and black—wasn't for her. "At that time, I didn't trust that instinct," she says, adding that she later learned to trust her instincts for what would make her comfortable in leadership settings.

A very successful nurse executive and elected policy maker, GLHS participant Nancy Valentine, Ph.D., R.N., described a dinner hosting a final candidate for a top position in a national health care organization. Although she liked the woman personally, she realized immediately that her expensive designer outfit would not communicate the appropriate message in this organization. "Unfortunately, it type-cast her," says Valentine, "and it reflected poorly on her ability to see that. I knew that judgment would be made by someone on the assessing team, and it was." She advises that women seek coaching and mentoring so they can be clear about what messages they want their appearance to convey.

Conversation Aids Effective Communication

The need to address communication barriers is critical in all health care contexts, not just leadership settings. Conversation is another form of presentation that can be an effective tool for productivity and generativity among groups and individuals who might otherwise remain apart. Conversation is a core business process, according to Juanita Brown, David Isaacs, and others who write for the Systems Thinker (1996). They work from the premise that conversing in professional settings and related networks catalyzes action. They have interviewed hundreds of executives in diverse cultures around the globe, and they find these recurring themes arising from conversation judged to be worthwhile in workplaces:

- A sense of mutual respect

- Taking time to talk with one another and reflect on what each thought was important

- Listening to each other, even when there are differences

- Being accepted and not judged by the others

- Strengthening the relationship through conversation

- Exploring important questions

- Developing a shared sense of meaning

- Learning something new and important

These findings may be critical to health care organizations as they compete in the knowledge economy (Webber, 1993, p. 24), because in these conversations, colleagues refine their ideas and thinking to create products and services. These dialogues lend themselves to clear, relevant, and thoughtful questions that set the stage for learning. From them, communities of practice often form, as we saw in Part One. These are groups that are formally and informally constructed, that operate with voluntary as well as positional input, and that are partnerlike in nature. Many such examples are emerging in health care—one is the Center for Nursing Leadership, originally sponsored by the Hill-Rom Corporation, the American Organization of Nurse Executives, and the Network for Healthcare Management. The Center is a vital web of individuals connected by an evolving collective intent based on shared values. Its members, geographically dispersed throughout the world, are connected centrally by computers. Seasonal face-to-face gatherings enhance their virtual link.

Dialogue Is Yet Another Tool

For many people, dialogue's timeless, agendaless process can be frustrating and arouse anxiety for those who are more action oriented. Yet it can allow us to get beyond knee-jerk reactions and hurling ideas at one another. Too often the goal of conversation is to reach a conclusion and to have one's views "win out" and be accepted by the group (Neuhauser, 1993, p. 53). Dialogue's proponents, on the other hand, call for participants' willingness, suspension of judgment, and allowing a sense of safety for those involved. Dialogue also plays an important role in effective leadership. The capacity for emotional expressiveness is a key ingredient in leadership purpose, persuasion, and inspiration, and dialogue helps achieve and demonstrate that expressiveness (Cooper and Sawaf, 1997, p. 68).

The Age-Old Communication: Storytelling

"There is no story until there is a telling" (Taylor, 1996). As we saw in Chapter Two, tribal behavior, gossip, and storytelling are the lifeblood of organizations. Gossip alone has had three functions historically: it provides information; it is a form of social control, influence, or entertainment; and it is used in socializing some professions, including nursing (Laing, 1993, pp. 37–43). Gossip can also be used as a weapon—it can sabotage a coworker's advancement or standing, as Duff describes in *When Women Work Together* (1993). It is also an excellent clue about the organization's culture. Listen to the current stories and gossip floating around a group or an institution, and you can produce an accurate diagnosis of that culture's characteristics.

Knowing and telling stories is an especially potent leadership skill in diverse health care settings. Leaders in vibrant cultures take responsibility for setting the tone—they encourage positive storytelling that includes building organizational heroes and heroines (Dreachslin, 1996, p. xi). Leland Kaiser, Ph.D., believes health care leaders are "going to reinvent everything, including our institutions. We are all storytellers—and the stories we tell create the reality in which we live."

An expert on organizational culture, author Peg Neuhauser believes that storytelling is the single most powerful form of human communication, and that stories about heroes are among the most important types of stories in organizations. We move so fast in health care organizational life that we often do not create time or place for storytelling. Neuhauser (1993) tells us that these stories represent the best of who we are, that they are our "sacred bundles" and that losing access to people's personal stories means losing portions of their wisdom, passion, and even heroism. We can afford to squander none of these things.

Neuhauser describes six types of positive stories that have special uses in health care:

1. *Hero stories:* The essence of the hero is the ability to live from the heart and to be human.

2. *Survivor stories:* Everything went wrong and we fixed it.

3. *Steam-valve stories:* The teller can vent, and others can respond. They help reduce stress and they build affinity. They can also be quite funny.

4. *Aren't-we-great stories:* We have reasons to be proud, enthusiastic, and even exaggerate if we feel like it.

5. *We-know-the-ropes-around-here stories:* These build culture and tribes.

6. *Kick-in-the-pants stories:* These are stories that motivate when they are well told.

Neuhauser offers simple suggestions for would-be storytellers: keep the plot short and simple, make the characters interesting and fun, use lots of action, keep the stories short, and rehearse to give yourself practice (Neuhauser, 1993, pp. 34–36).

William G. Gonzalez described a storytelling experience of immeasurable value to his organization. He had noticed that staff would ask people if they needed help finding their way around the hospital buildings—even if they weren't lost–and he noticed that the "heroes" were often women. So he established a program called "Make a Difference." If someone reported an act of kindness, the person who offered the kindness received a coupon for $1 off in the cafeteria. At first twenty or thirty names were submitted, then fifty or sixty. He invited a number of employees—members of the housekeeping staff would come in suits and ties—into the boardroom each month to have coffee with him, and he asked them to describe in their own words what they had done. "The stories would just knock your socks off!" says Gonzalez. "In many cases it was the women that were most comfortable telling the story. They were also best at expressing and seeing or helping those who were confused, lost or in grief." He adds that men could see those stumbling around and obviously lost, but the women could also see others who were more subtly in need.

Changing Communication's Cadence

A number of GLHS contributors, whose positions range from health system chief executive officers to senior government leaders and prominent academicians, offer women (and men) tips for communicating well:

- David Kindig, M.D., Ph.D.: "Be straight. Communicate with clarity, precision, and directness. Often we play communication games for ourselves, not for others."

- Maura Fields, R.N.: "I really enjoy listening to people, for often I am able to hear what is *not* being said. Therefore I have more information that helps me make decisions." But proceed with caution. Eunice Azzani warns of a surprising constraint on listening well—our own enthusiasm and passion when it gets in the way of hearing the other's message.

- The late Duayne Walker, R.N.: "If you say something as a health care leader, whether it be a principal or a value, your behavior must show your values."

- Nando Zepeda, M.P.H.: "Lives are at risk. Pull your ego out of it."

- Linda Burnes Bolton, Ph.D., R.N.: "Effective communication requires that you learn about who you are talking with. Every time I check in with a group, I ask 'why you are here? Are we meeting your goals?'"

- David Fine, M.H.A.: "Particularly when an organization is going through a lot of change, over-communicating is necessary. One cannot assume that the chain of command works."

- Sister Mary Jean Ryan: "Effective communication doesn't mean lots of communication. It means timely communication, identifying the important matters, communicating succinctly. In other words, don't take up my whole day."

- Hudson Birden, M.P.H.: "The leader must be able to think on her feet. She must have all the knowledge 'right there.' If it's not, defer in order to reflect and research. A lawyer put Henry Ford on a witness stand and tried to make him look stupid by quizzing him on minutia of auto manufacture. Ford won the day by responding that he didn't need to keep that knowledge in his head when he knew how to look up in five minutes!"

Summing Up

This chapter reviews key socialization and communication differences between men and women in leadership roles in health care, and how these differences can be perceived. It also summarizes the GLHS contributors' techniques for more effective presentation strategies for women—including those that are nonverbal.

From here we move to Chapter Seven, which focuses on career renewal strategies and how to employ them in service of our professional commitments.

7

Antidote 3: Career Renewal Strategies

I magine yourself in a rink trying to control a bumper car as other cars sideswipe you at many turns—turns taking you in directions you never intended. This experience is very like that of most health care leaders, particularly women, whose careers seldom progress in a linear fashion. Instead, they move in what GLHS contributor Karen Ehrat describes as the "bumper theory of career progress." Many of us seemingly ricochet from one opportunity, choice, or circumstance to another. But there's no need for embarrassment. Indeed, women (and men) can take solace in research findings across many industries, including health care, that career progression for most women is not a methodical "rise to power" but a zigzag course of ups, downs, and plateaus (Aburdene and Naisbitt, 1992, p. 48).

Women take advantage of the opportunities available to them while balancing the family circumstances that demand their attention. Indeed, well-known health care executive recruiter Peter Rabinowitz believes that it is just this intricacy of women's lives that uniquely qualifies them to serve as leaders. They are the ultimate jugglers and arbiters—of work, home, family, and self—and they bring this capacity to top leadership roles. Because it is the leader's job to allocate scarce resources among competing demands, who better for the job than the female who has been doing this all her adult life?

Women's careers are an accumulation of experiences that Association of American Medical Colleges vice president Janet Bickel dubs "accumulating advantages and disadvantages." Although she specifically cites women in academic medicine, her concept applies across health care settings. When thinking in terms of accumulating advantages and disadvantages, the career picture, and the skills women bring to their chosen leadership arena, women's careers are always works in progress. A given point in time is not the result of one set of factors, but many that collect over time (Friedman, 1994).

This chapter offers a variety of options, based largely on GLHS contributor's suggestions, for mitigating career disadvantages and enhancing advantages. We explore the following:

- What health care leadership careers may encompass in the future

- What women can do to manage the glass ceilings they encounter

- How women (and men) can develop and evaluate their own skills and personal characteristics to attain their career and leadership goals

- Learning and its relationship to leadership effectiveness at all stages and places in the health care spectrum

Health Care Careers and Leadership in the Future

Many prognosticators believe that providing health care will increasingly fall to women. But in what context will this occur? What will the health care system consist of? Futurist Leland R. Kaiser has long proposed that the imminent health care system will be a key factor in the emerging cultural focus on human growth and development. He terms this phenomenon "human potentiation"— which, according to him, will be the future's biggest business.

In the meantime, today's health care organizations continue to transform at a rapid pace as they adjust to managing the health of populations, rather than just the diseases of individuals. Wanda Jones, among others, predicts that this level of transformation will last at least two decades. Whatever the shape and structure of health care in the new century, consumer interest in healing will only increase. Some health care organizations will move aggressively into this area while maintaining their traditional focus on medical care. The community will offer many opportunities for healing at schools, churches, workplaces, sports events, street ministries, homeless shelters, senior apartments, and the like. These have certain advantages for health care providers, including out-of-pocket payment, volunteer help, using others' space, increased market visibility, and even increased trust (Jones, 1997).

Although the future may hold career opportunities that mitigate current gender barriers, many women today continue to work in traditionally structured and focused organizations. Some women are being elevated to the top spots, but others are being promoted to what *used to be* the top spots, according to a study contributor who observes industry trends nationwide. "Women outlast their male counterparts who lose their jobs during downsizing or mergers," this contributor says. "They are then promoted to the top institutional position, which is often downgraded from CEO to COO. The new organization gets an experienced executive, who is expected to be relatively compliant with a new regime, cost less, and bring less promotion ambition for the top system job."

Managing That Glass Ceiling

Clearly, many women and men are concerned about paving a smoother path for women so they may draw out needed talent for their organizations. In 1991, *Hospitals* magazine convened a series of experts to address how the "glass ceiling" in health care can be "shattered." They emerged with suggestions that still apply today.

1. *Gatekeepers—CEOs and others—must actively groom women for top-level positions.* Most GLHS contributors lamented the absence of time for being either a mentee or a mentor. But these relationships are critical for all would-be leaders, as well as for the leaders themselves. Without grooming for the top jobs, no one, regardless of sex, can succeed.

2. *Women will have to make personal trade-offs.* Of course, this is not news to any woman who has ever considered a leadership position.

3. *Women must learn to aim high in their career aspirations.* Despite the ambivalence many women experience about making family and personal sacrifices to pursue the top jobs, they must assess their readiness to commit to moving ahead. Also, the organizations of which they are part must assist them as they prepare and assume these posts.

4. *Women must work on self-esteem issues, convince themselves they have the skills, and gain more responsible jobs* (Eubanks, 1991). Key to women's collective ability to move into the highest levels of management are preparing themselves for the barriers to success while not being overtaken by them; augmenting their own skills and strategies; and developing strong and empowering beliefs about themselves. Self-esteem is critical, as we saw in Chapter Four.

Harvard Business School professor Rosabeth Moss Kanter has long studied organizational behavior and its impact on women. As early as 1977, she observed what is still true today: "Women must rely on themselves rather than on institutions to create [their] careers. They must be entrepreneurs who make their own opportunities—either within or outside a major corporation—or professionals with portable career assets—skills and reputations that can be applied anywhere" (Kanter, 1977, p. 272).

New Approaches to Work and "The Job"

Many women, and some men too, require accommodation to manage the many components of their lives, particularly during their parenting years.

Flexible Job Structure

A number of GLHS contributors believe that women simply cannot "have it all" at the most senior levels, at least not all at the same time, particularly if they are parenting young children. We have also seen that a key limitation is our singular *model* of leadership. When there is an opportunity for reorganization or recruitment, boards and senior staff will do well to seriously question the assumption that all senior positions must be full-time and assumed by a single individual.

Today's tradition in many health care organizations requires this format, yet it severely limits the pool of female candidates for top jobs. Many such women are competent and willing to serve if their needs as active parents can be accommodated—at least for a few years. Shared leadership models are working successfully in high-technology industries as well as other entrepreneurial ventures, and they can be successfully adopted in health care, too.

Everyone loses when flexibility isn't even considered. One interviewee, for example, commented on her attempt to develop a shared leadership post in a small organization. When personal circumstances required her to renegotiate her CEO role from full to part time, she proposed dividing the position so she could focus her well-acknowledged efforts on what she did best—bringing in new business. She suggested engaging someone else to manage the business that was already in place, and offered a way to contain expense and provide financial incentives for this arrangement. "The answer was a swift 'no way,'" she recalls. "I was to be the full-time CEO, something 'lesser,' or nothing at all. My circumstances and their lack of willingness to consider an alternative made my choice obvious: I chose nothing at all."

Fortunately, this narrow exercise of options will become less common, at least in many organizations. Virtual communication systems are providing viable platforms for women and men to augment their presence on the job by working from remote locations, including their homes or even other parts of the country.

Own Your Career

You will never own your job, but you do own your career. GLHS contributor Eunice Azzani, a career management expert and successful recruiter in not-for-profit organizations, watches the sometimes circuitous path to leadership for women. Her advice to women who would be leaders at the highest levels: "Here's how to think about your career: 'I am the product. Now, what would I like to do with it?'"

Azzani believes this is the decade, even the millennium, of the woman. As women take charge of their careers and assert themselves as responsible stewards of health care organizations, systems, and communities, she encourages them to do so without the sense of "entitlement" that some women now display. Instead, she and other GLHS contributors urge that the emotional force for their career choices well up from renewed passion, purpose, and commitment.

Know your assets, know how to be a catalyst for action, and tell your stories, advises Azzani, who encourages women to reflect on any career situation they are considering by asking, "Do I add value? What is it? Will I receive value?" Finally, she reminds women that they should not assume change can be made incrementally: "Sometimes the envelope must be pushed."

Rethinking "The Job"

In his important book *Jobshift: How to Prosper in a Workplace Without Jobs* (1995), William Bridges was the first of several authors to cut new ground. The traditional job—that vehicle that has carried our productivity at work—is going away because the kind of work, the terms of work, and the unit of work are changing fundamentally.

As a consequence, we will have to create new work realities, such as compensation plans, work profiles, measures of performance, policies and forms of job sharing, communication policies, and organizational structures. Key to Bridges's assessment is that traditional jobs aren't very flexible, as we have just seen, and that they will not lend themselves to this complex and changing environment.

These predictions, now spreading across many industries, have important ramifications on career development for women in health care. The generation of women who usher in the millennium will be the first workers who are "free agents," finding themselves in a world of constant opportunity and stiff competition. To manage this successfully, Bridges advises individuals to forget "coping" with change. To cope would be reactive. Instead, they must make these changes work *for* them. Organizations too must build flexibility into their structures, policies, training programs, and strategies (Bridges, 1994).

Reevaluate and Develop Discrete, Interchangable Skills

Promoting and taking advantage of the increasingly flexible leadership marketplace requires having a clear and objective view of the skills we offer. Developing fresh vision about these skills includes seeing them as component parts that can be rearranged to fit specific needs. This viewpoint frees us to serve as autonomous agents even when we are in full-time jobs. With this philosophy, we implement Azzani's statement: we are a "product." What we bring to any leadership context is our package of services—a unique set of assets, or "product" that is customized to fill the singular needs of the buyer.

Gail Sheehy, the prolific author who has studied life cycles of men and women in modern society, provides additional perspective: "A single fixed identity is a liability today. It only makes people more vulnerable to sudden changes in economic or personal conditions. The most successful and healthy among us now develop 'multiple identities,' managed simultaneously, to be called upon as conditions change" (Sheehy, 1995, p. 71).

Career Mapping

Having portable skills is critically important in health care, as in many other fields. Career mapping can help. This can be an elaborate step-by-step process or a simple exercise in which the leader identifies the essence of her skills and then tries out the fit between those skills and different contexts. Discussing the questions with someone else is most effective—but even a few hours of brainstorming solo can yield new possibilities. These key inquiries will get you started:

What is your personal vision for yourself? What is your ideal "job" or work situation?

Where do elements of your dream setting exist today? What can you do to learn more about these opportunities?

Where and how *do* you add value? Where and how *can* you add value?

What's your core body of knowledge? How does your package of knowledge, skills, motivations, and desires fit with the opportunities in or outside your organization? Think expansively, brainstorm, and don't eliminate any idea in the first phase because it doesn't seem realistic.

What's your gift? Don't worry if it is like someone else's—that doesn't matter. Your unique combination of skills, abilities, experience, interests, and commitments is the base from which you will best serve others, and yourself.

What brings you joy and inspires your highest quality efforts and your greatest contribution?

What do you want to learn? What do you want to teach? These answers give you important clues about the most vital future for yourself.

Who do you want to work with? Why? Are these individuals from whom you will learn, by whom you will be respected, and with whom you will enjoy making the contribution that is most important to you?

Embrace Your Uniqueness

A pattern emerged early in my interviews for the GLHS: several individuals who have had major national impact through their authorial, policy, and health system leadership voices consider themselves to be outside the norm, even "marginal" in some way. Their statements in the interviews were not veiled compliments to their own "genius." Rather, they reflected an almost self-conscious admission that their intellect, leadership prowess, or skills were not valued in the mainstream early in their careers.

Today, these fully mature but still unusual qualities flower in their bearers, bringing them increasing opportunities for impact and great national regard. They have spent years honing and successfully focusing these talents. Yet many of these individuals still consider themselves different. Today, their distinctions can range from not partaking of business dinners, to shunning operational responsibility and the chance to move up, to never having been strong working inside an organization. They also include maintaining family or religious boundaries at the expense of traditional executive behavior, such as working on weekends.

What is important about these choices is that each of these individuals is successful *as a result of* valuing and developing her own talents, even if they were not understood or judged as important early on. Today, these same people continue to stay true to their chosen values and primary commitments even in the face of great professional pressure to do otherwise.

The first example of this phenomenon was offered by an international health care expert. In the interview, he rather shyly described a recent prespeech introduction from a business icon that he had always respected. His colleague had lovingly referred to him as a "marginal man," meaning he "didn't quite 'fit in'."

This anecdote was followed by another from a woman—a near icon herself—who created her own business some years ago. Keenly aware of differences between herself and other health care leaders at that time, she says she chose a career path that was unusual so her differences could shine. Those differences included a highly focused perspective about the ways health care can best be provided, as well as a perception that she can be more effective by being on the outside rather than the inside of traditional organizations.

Still another nationally regarded female contributor recounted that early in her career she had been told after a week of leadership training that she would never be a leader. Since that time fifteen years ago, she has gone on to influence health care policy and operations from a position of national stature. Rather than take the early feedback as a prediction of doom, she used it to form her goals for continued development.

Women and men who question their leadership potential, or have had it questioned by others, can take heart. They can also take action, as many of the study contributors did, by using the feedback they received to outline a course of continued learning. They also refused to take other's negative assessments as indictments—instead they used the information to focus their talents and bolster their skills to suit the roles they sought.

Factor in Forgiveness

Like most human beings, professionals oscillate between periods of greater and lesser success. GLHS contributor David Fine, Regents Professor and chairman of the School of Public Health at Tulane University Medical Center, is a former health system CEO. He calls for health care leaders to incorporate the quality of forgiveness as they evaluate leadership potential. "Everyone does not build a career from triumph to triumph," he says. "Sometimes it is important to pick people up, dust them off, and help them move on."

Live into the Future

David Bohm, a physicist who is best known as the father of "dialogue" as discussed in Chapter Six, offers helpful counsel through his words to a colleague who was struggling to control his career: "You cannot be fixed in how you're going about it any more than you would be fixed if you were setting about to paint a great work of art. Be alert, be self-aware, so that when opportunity presents itself, you can actually rise to it. . . . We are creating the future every moment" (Jaworski, 1996, p. 83).

Learning, Leadership, and Organizational Success

Time and again, GLHS contributors came back to the importance of continuing to learn. Acknowledging and acting upon this wisdom is crucial to meet the continuing demands for changed and socially responsible health care.

Individual commitment to renewed learning is most effective when it is accompanied by an organizational focus on learning, as well. There are real benefits for organizations that operationalize their stated beliefs about this principle. Chief among them is that organizational learning contributes to dynamic and consistent organizational culture. According to GLHS contributor Joel Shalowitz, M.D., of the Kellogg School at Northwestern University, one of the greatest single competitive advantages for an organization is such a culture: "We train people with tools, but then we pass on training them in 'what works.' People's skills are key, yet it is also important to create a consistent culture, mission, vision, focus, and team building. This is the critical competitive advantage."

If such commitment to regular personal and professional learning yields competitive advantage, its lack, according to one health care consultant who works with hundreds of CEOs throughout the United States, is "catastrophic." She predicts that health care organizations eventually will replace those employees who don't learn, because "their value erodes every day they do not enhance their wisdom and skills."

Learning Is a Continuing Cycle

Most seasoned professionals believe leaders learn, move up a notch in expertise and station, then learn again in a continual, progressive, linear movement. But in a knowledge economy, and in competency-based professions such as those in health care, learning is a continuing cycle of assessing and selectively accessing new information. It is also a process of emptying out. Learning is as much about relearning, or changing attitudes, habits, and beliefs that get in the way of achieving different results, as it is about taking in new information.

Robert D. Haas, longtime chairman and CEO of Levi Strauss & Co., puts it this way: "It's difficult to unlearn behaviors that made us successful in the past. Speaking rather than listening. Valuing people like yourself over people of a different gender or from different cultures. Doing things on your own rather than collaborating. Making the decision yourself instead of asking different people for their perspectives. There's a whole range of behaviors that were highly functional in the old hierarchical organization that are dead wrong in the flatter, more responsive empowered organization that we're seeking to become" (Bennis, 1996, pp. 259–260).

Leadership Is Synonymous with Learning

GLHS contributor Sandra Hernandez, M.D., says that "being effective as a health care leader has a direct correlation with the ability to learn. This is particularly true in big jobs, in which one's tendency is to be an inch thick and a mile wide." Her belief was echoed by two other contributors, both male CEOs of major health care concerns. One adds, "leadership *is* learning."

Willingness to Learn is a Predictor of Leadership Success

Contributor Robert Boyle, M.P.H., considers commitment to learning carefully as he hires others and evaluates new career opportunities for himself: "When I pick people to work with, I ask 'Is this individual a learning person? Has this person demonstrated adaptability?' These are also ways to 'size up' someone you're going to work for."

Learning Is a Survival Skill for Leaders—Literally

Two GLHS contributors, neither mincing words, made very similar comments. The first is from a female CEO: "If you're not learning, you're dead." The second is from a well-recognized leader in the national arena. She says, "If senior leaders don't learn, they will be canned eventually." The message: "Take a hard look at yourself and make corrections. It's important to recognize your own incompetence before someone else does."

Acknowledge Failure and Learn from It

Winston Churchill once said that success is going from failure to failure without a loss of enthusiasm (Cooper and Sawaf, 1997, p. 120). "Failures" teach us the art of falling. Chris Argyris, a noted professor and organization theorist at Harvard University Business School, observes many professionals who are almost always successful at what they do. Because they rarely experience failure, they have never learned how to learn from it. The result: they become defensive, screen out criticism, and put blame on everyone and everything except themselves. The leader's ability to learn shuts down precisely at the moment they need it the most (Argyris, 1991, p. 109).

Learning Means Acknowledging Problems

Managers' and leaders' continual upbeat behavior can actually inhibit learning. "Managers often censor what everyone needs to say and hear," says Argyris. "For the sake of 'morale' and 'considerateness,' they deprive employees and themselves of the opportunity to take responsibility for their own behavior by learning to understand it." When important organizational problems become potentially threatening, "rigorous reasoning goes right out the window and defensive reasoning takes over." This discourages reflection, and encourages a second level of defensiveness—organizationally defensive routines. "These consist of all the policies, practices, and actions that prevent human beings from having to experience embarrassment or threat, and at the same time, prevent them from examining the nature and causes of that embarrassment or threat," (Argyris, 1991, pp. 99–109).

Practice Makes Perfect

According to author Traci Goss (1996, p. 198), practice gives an individual "absolute ownership of the field. In any field, being extraordinary requires a form of practice in which there is constant reexamination of all that's come before; in which she who practices lets go of everything that has worked before and creates a new future whenever it is needed. Practice is the determining distinction between the novice and the master."

Leaders Learn Through Feedback

The day I interviewed one highly experienced male executive, he had been given a coveted award by his colleagues from around the country. Despite this admiration and success (or because of them), he says he is always open to ways to improve himself and cites a recent example of several senior people who told him that he often appeared distracted in meetings. "Feedback is still a source of my professional growth," he says. "I learned greatly from their candor and trust."

Learning Turns on Reflection

One GLHS contributor described how, ten years ago, she learned the value of reflection. "The CEO told me that I needed to use my 'feminine wiles'—and that I was too straightforward," she says. "At first I was angry and insulted. Then I sorted through what it was the CEO was trying to tell me, concluding that it is not always good to have a ready answer. One should listen and reflect first and then determine the appropriate response to get the desired outcome. I have seen both men and women use this technique successfully."

Point/Counterpoint

How do males and females compare as they approach their learning and career opportunities in health care? What can we learn from one another to bolster our chances for greater success? The views of the GLHS contributors are instructive.

Advice About and from Male Leaders in Health Care

"Men are willing to make compacts with each other. They support each other in ways that count. Women do not do that. They are still trying to break through to their own power base. Men are also skilled at waiting their turn, and then acting."—Barbara Donaho, R.N., M.A.

Men are more career focused in their networking relationships. "They are more purposeful than women in their networking, and they stay focused on an expected or perceived outcome, such as getting a better job. Women's reasons for networking are more affiliative, supportive, to get feedback, for confirmation of self, fun and building self-esteem."—Nancy Valentine, Ph.D., R.N.

Is good career strategy second nature for men? A significant number of women ascribed well-honed career management skills to men. Yet at least two career-savvy men provide insight into their "second nature." A mid-career CEO of a major health system with a history of top positions volunteered that his career is the "second or last thing I am doing [strategizing] at any given time." The second male, who has had an equally impressive string of key positions, doesn't focus on this either. But he says that he makes sure when he takes on a new job that he doesn't follow superstars. He adds that in a new job, he sits and listens at least three months: "I also ask 'if you were in my position, what would you do?' I write down their answers and see what comes up repeatedly."

Know thyself. A successful male in his mid-forties undergoing an intense career challenge distinguished between knowledge of the field and how to do his job. He speaks metaphorically, from his musical success with his off-hours band: "I know I won't be a great bass player, for example, but I know how to compensate and be as good as I can in an actual playing situation. That's important."

Know when to fold 'em. One male senior vice president offers this advice: "It is important to recognize when you need to move on. At my last position, I was the most senior person on the team and I knew they would 'get me' eventually. I had too much power. It's important to step outside of yourself and look at the need for new motivations for yourself." In fact, says JoEllen Koerner, Ph.D., R.N., "work your way out of your job." In other words, do the work you came to do, then move on to your next chosen endeavor.

Success is not always moving up. One male, who has also moved successfully within high-ranking positions throughout the country, doesn't link those moves to more money. "It's been important for me to realize you can change jobs and make less money," he says. "I'm happier, having followed what I want to do."

Preempt a midlife crisis. David J. Fine has held several CEO positions and is now a professor. He is thoughtful about the midlife transition that can plague men and women in their middle years. "The symptoms range from people getting tired of working; feeling unfulfilled in their careers; marriages collapsing; too much drinking, etc.," he notes. "I have taken preemptive strikes by assuring that one year in my career hasn't looked like the next. Every three to five years, I make a major change. Most recently I chose to leave line operations for teaching and research—at age 47."

Advice to Women from Women

Don't blame men. "I am sick of blaming doctors, hospitals, men, and women" exclaimed one female in considering women's leadership opportunities. "It's far better to ask 'what exists,' 'how do I fix it,' and 'what do I do to get there?'"

Stay in tune. "Listen, read, grab the 'thread' of what's going on around you," urges Polly Bednash, Ph.D., executive director of the American Association of Colleges of Nursing. "You must stay knowledgeable about the world. You need to have a finger on a lot of pulses. Although it can be frustrating, you must be willing to do this to be a good leader."

Flexibility and competence are key tools. Professor of management at San Diego State University School of Public Health, Alma Koch has held key leadership positions in large managed care entities. She and several others relate to the bumper car theory of career progress mentioned earlier. Strategies are great, says Koch, but adds that such career management is not possible given the changes in the today's health care environment. "The key is flexibility—there are all kinds of opportunities—don't start dwelling on just one," she advises.

Be careful about what you become good at doing. Elaina Genser cautions women to be open to new things, but careful about how long they do them. "It is good to be a utility in-field player, but you don't want to be left there," she warns. "If you do some cleanup, you may suddenly get stuck there, e.g., in human resources. If you are too good at it, you can get sidelined." Instead, she counsels women to build up their resumes by volunteering or going on to a new project, adding that it is important to get exposure, maybe in the lead role, perhaps as a "consultant de facto" working with a board or something similar.

Think long term. What impact do you want to have? One accomplished female urges women to stop focusing on gender limitations and get to the values and traits we want to *see* in each other and the career options we want to *have*. For example, go on to become a great consultant if it's not possible to succeed as a leader within a conservative institution. At least one GLHS contributor has elected that course for her career. Also, if you want something, go for it, a strategy Elaine Cohen, Ph.D., R.N., noted expert on case management, has always used: "I went into nursing and nursing leadership with the idea that I was going to contribute. I have been clear about what I wanted, and 'they' have all said 'yes!' I did not resonate with all people, of course, but those I did resonate with have come to my rescue."

Create the antidote to the "job in a box." Cohen's career exemplifies what Moss Kanter and others have implored women to do: create their own careers. Cohen has always envisioned a parallel professional life in addition to her paid positions: writing with consulting on the side. "I had done the traditional 9-to-5 route, having my passion on the side. I kept 'doing' and 'doing,' and all of a sudden, I had something else to fall back on," she says. GLHS contributor and managed care expert Connie Burgess's career is similar. As a successful independent consultant, she always knew she wanted to have her own business, and ten years ago she decided to take the leap. (Details on how she accomplished this are in Chapter Ten.)

Use your life patterns, challenges, and successes. One study contributor, an accomplished female nurse executive who has demonstrated leadership skills all her life, is now a key leader with a very large national organization. She has also undergone a serious illness and protracted personal experience in the health care system. Now, she says, "I am *very* committed to clinical improvement." She is very vocal and effective in expressing this commitment in her high-impact role.

Make hard choices. GLHS contributor Pam Thompson's singular career success as a senior nurse executive in New Hampshire has required her to make difficult choices, as she is a leader in both nursing and administration. "I am vice president for three services. I am the chief nurse and I am also the administrator," she explains. "People attribute to me that I am a nurse first—and this is perceived to be a conflict of interest, according to some. At times, I feel their perceptions do not allow me to be one or the other."

Be choosy. When Sandra Hernandez was graduated from medical school, a mentor advised her: don't ever take a job you don't want to do. During most of her searches for new positions, Hernandez has written out the ideals she associates with her next job, and in most cases has accepted positions that match the ideal. "The three criteria I use are: the quality of the contribution I can make; the learning I can acquire, and the level of resistance to what I will be trying to achieve in the position," she says.

Summing Up

This chapter focuses on key career strategies and ways women and men can learn from one another's successes. The next chapter highlights the need for learning in a different context—personal renewal for the leader herself and professional renewal and learning through mentoring those around her.

8

Antidote 4: Nurturing Ourselves, Mentoring Others

Section One: Self-Renewal

"That fire, which should be burning so bright inside you, is consuming rather than warming you" (Feudenberger, 1980, p. 210). All too often, this lament describes what is happening to many health care leaders—the committed, yet exhausted, stewards of their own and others' health. Here we come face to face with another paradox. Excited about seeing the word "renewal" on the survey and quick to confirm that renewal is important, even critical, the GLHS contributors say the chances for renewal just aren't there—once again presenting a gap between the real and the ideal.

This chapter offers a variety of viewpoints, inspiring comments, and options for renewal—a key leadership need that too often goes unhonored. We explore what personal and professional renewal is, why we need it, why we don't do it, and realistic alternatives for bringing it into our professional lives. Connected to renewal is mentoring, and we will discuss what that is, how it can be practiced differently, and how this process benefits us as both mentors and leaders. Because health care is about healing the sick and promoting the well-being and care of others, our leaders are, at least intellectually, aware of the importance of regeneration. Few if any have to be reminded of the body's requirement for rest, the psyche's need for refreshment, or our overall need for sustenance at many levels. Self-renewal, as one interviewee put it, is "an absolute must for anyone who is ambitious—whatever renewal is for you, whether it be taking

a nap or running a triathlon, is the most important element of finding balance in life."

Martial arts expert Frank Rivers sees renewal as creating a "space"
that becomes the leader's platform, from which she *chooses* her actions
rather than just reacting to circumstances confronting her. When she
simply reacts, she falls back on outmoded, ingrained habits. In *The
Way of the Owl* (1996), Rivers likens this subtle dimming of consciousness to not knowing the difference between the map and the
territory. "Reality is dynamic and yet our vocabularies change slowly,
if at all," he writes. Professional and leadership habits change just as
slowly unless we take steps to reflect and renew ourselves.

Actions Belie Belief

Let's explore why we are not good at matching our behavior with
our belief in renewal. One contributor, an executive recruiter in
contact with many senior leaders nationally, talks about the people
she sees "burning out," who want to go back in time or escape to
wherever there is less managed care. "People take no vacations and
they cannot get away," she says.

She also sheds light on the absence of women in visible leadership roles. Without time off, "How can people handle their own
lives, let alone the extra dimension of outside organizational leadership, and the time involved in going through all the 'chairs' so
they can assume the key positions?" While adding that the irony is
their effectiveness increases after they have taken time off, she
attributes part of the prevailing trend to the lack of training positions: "People go from manager to director to vice president. There
is no place to mentor, train and do *part*, but *not all*, of the job."

GLHS contributor Pam Thompson, who calls the lack of opportunity for renewal "one of the greatest paradoxes of our profession,"
worries about another of its consequences: "I see everybody going
crazy—and this is gender-neutral. The younger people don't want
to step into our roles."

There may be other serious costs as well. In their best-selling book *Built to Last: Successful Habits of Visionary Companies* (1994), James C. Collins and Jerry L. Porras report the results of their study of companies that sustain their quality over time. Self-renewal was one of the most important aspects for these highly successful, enduring businesses. Flourishing companies offer sabbatical programs, continuing education opportunities, flexible work schedules, telecommuting options, and a variety of other employee-driven programs designed to revitalize the employees and the company itself. Health care organizations must pay attention to this. Says one GLHS contributing CEO: "The 'whine quotient' is high in health care management, because executives tire, lose their edge, and don't refresh themselves." As does Thompson, he sees the problem as gender-neutral.

In Chapter Two, Blue Cross/Blue Shield president and CEO Patrick Hays talked about his experience leading an organization that took so much pride in the dedication of its executives that it inadvertently put off women from seeking top leadership roles. In some health care companies, such pride translates into routine fifty- and sixty-hour workweeks. When executives consciously or unconsciously perpetuate cultures that require themselves, as well those with whom they work, to work long hours each day, each week, and each month, even the best system and its managers suffer. Thus evolves a vicious cycle of degeneration. Declining productivity ensues as individuals caught within the system act as if more effort and time on the job will produce more gain, even though they know rationally that *amount* of effort does not equal *quality* of outcome.

At its core, self-renewal is simply allowing for a cycle of change that includes resting, learning, and growing. Significant for executives, it permits time to be open, even naïve or unsure, much as leaders taking on new tasks or positions must be. A new job demands renewal, requiring leaders of each sex to bear with the uncomfortable feelings of not knowing whether they are on course in an unfamiliar situation. This calls for a different leadership competency: the ability to "succeed at following" (Frantz and Pattakos, 1996, p. 78).

Forms of Renewal

The author of several books on healing, Joan Borysenko, Ph.D., reminds us that rejuvenation comes in many forms, particularly for women, and it may arrive as success, relationships, or a feeling of balance. Her own life is an example: her literary success has created heavy demands on her professional and personal time. She finds that at times she is the target of near-pity about this intense period in her life. But she believes that busy lives are not necessarily unhappy lives, backing up her statement with research from the Wellesley College Center for Research on Women. The Center's Lifeprints Study found that "One of the main pleasures of busy working women . . . is the relatively large number of relationships . . . they maintain." She practices what she calls inner balance. "When I am in balance, what the Navajos call walking in beauty, I naturally think of the results of my actions," she says. "I am most creative, in harmony with my work. Everything gets done more elegantly, simply, and efficiently because a greater wisdom inspires my thoughts and actions" (Borysenko, 1996, pp. 135–138).

Renewal for leaders can arrive somewhat masked within the term "transitional incompetence." This state occurs when new skills are required but not yet attained, such as computer skills to access information remotely. Or it can apply to those dangerous, fragile periods when, having changed jobs, for example, leaders are visible and responsible in new ways. For men, these situations can be particularly fraught as many have been taught to appear competent in all situations, as we saw in Chapter Four.

Women face different challenges: while practicing the skills that will establish perceptions of competence, they must also be permitted perceptions of "incompetence" from time to time. They need freedom to ask what they do not know and to seek opinions to inform their own without being viewed as less than fully capable. Allowing for and even encouraging transitional incompetence is crucial for growth and development. In Chapter Seven, one GLHS contributor explained that he spends the first three months of a new job listening. Doing this gives him time to exist in, and then move beyond, transitional incompetence.

Many GLHS contributors offered inspiring, if not universally practiced, views of how health care executives, irrespective of gender, can view and implement renewal:

Renewal as Lifelong Learning. For Nando Zepeda, now retired senior health executive of the Los Angeles County Department of Health, renewal is like lifelong learning. "It starts with the lowest level—personal renewal must occur in order for there to be organizational renewal," he says. "Small health care organizations and the people who are integrated into their activities do practice this. Beehives self-renew—so too do people."

Renewal as Sharing Successes and Feedback. A nursing leader in a large organization talks with staff nurses and asks them to share their positive experiences. A female CEO who sets time aside for evaluation, retreats, and the like invites "360-degree" evaluations in a manner in which people feel safe. "This is never easy for me, but I do it." A male academic volunteers to do new things: "For the advanced executive, learning to say no *and* to say yes selectively is key. We constantly hear to learn to say no, but leaders also need to look for opportunities to help them grow."

Renewal as Balance. For a number of survey respondents, renewal comes from personal balance. GLHS contributor Maura Fields is a nurse executive and key member of the management team at North Valley Hospital in Whitefish, Montana. Fields says balance is "the point between strength and power—which we assign to men—and vulnerability—which we assign to women. In balance, it is perfect. For example, if a woman is strong in a white male system, men *and* women are discouraged in fragility and vulnerability." For others, balance is maintaining space between the personal and the professional life. The late Duane D. Walker, R.N., M.S., F.A.A.N., former vice president of patient services at the Queen's Medical Center in Honolulu, Hawaii, set limits that enabled him to observe his personal commitment to balance. Those limits included not accepting speaking engagements for Saturday or Sunday, not attending local weekend workshops, and only attending weekend work or work-social functions when he really wanted to. He took frequent brief vacations, had many hobbies and, except for four or five times a year, made sure he did not take work home.

Renewal as Self-Confidence. One successful contributor offers another perspective for those who just work harder and harder: "I was talking with a colleague whom I respect about a coworker who worked eighty hours a week, and the colleague said, 'Maybe so-and-so is a poor organizer.'" She continued, "This statement allowed me to see a truth about many leaders I know, many of whom see themselves as 'victims,' because of the demands of their schedules." She questions why people work this hard: "Do they fear losing power? I don't fear this. I am respected and I also believe that if I am going to lose my job, I won't prevent it by being here eighteen hours a day."

Renewal as Self-Love. Nancy Valentine believes that renewal begins with self-love. "We can't practice self-renewal without love for ourselves, and it can be done in a million small ways. For example, I recently bought a small sculptured incense burner. When I light the incense, I feel rejuvenated. It helps me sleep 'like a baby!'"

Renewal as Consciousness. GLHS contributor Cathy Michaels looks to ancient ways to self-renew, such as meditation, looking at the whole of things, exercising, and being in nature. "I have learned the difference between being 'done' and being 'finished for now,'" she says.

Renewal as Presence. Slowing down and living in the present allows us to see aspects of our life that were "previously hidden in the frenzy of a busy mind and hectic schedule," counsels contributor and retired Navy captain Jane Swanson, R.N.

Creating the Space for Restoration

Author Mihaly Csikszentmihalyi believes that giving people advice about renewal is useless, "Because they already have too many demands on their time and they 'can't afford to do anything new or interesting.'" However, he does believe it is important to question how we spend our time and to husband it accordingly. Time is what we must find in order to enjoy life, and the other important renewal resource is the "ability to control psychic energy. To control attention means to control experience, and therefore the quality of life." (Csikszentmihalyi, 1990, p. 127).

As do some GLHS contributors, authors and consultants Cooper and Sawaf distinguish between identifying "big" renewal activities, such as a trip or weekend away, and the ability to see a renewal opportunity, no matter how small. What's important is "learning to choose the most appropriate [renewal option] on the spot, and to catch and turn around downsliding energy or mood. It's up to each of us to identify practical skills to stay more adaptable whenever we get our backs up, or start feeling tense or tired, to renew ourselves regularly along the way" (Cooper and Sawaf, 1997, p. 126).

Does Gender Affect Renewal?

Many GLHS contributors who lamented the cycle of too much work and too little time attributed some of these problems to gender. A nurse executive on sabbatical during the time of her interview said that what she was doing was unusual. She feels that men are better at taking time off. "Men will take the day off if a friend comes to town, often without consulting a calendar to see what is occurring," she says. "But women need to be the best of everything, do the right thing. We will cancel or delay vacations, come back early from a vacation—we will sacrifice what we need to do for ourselves."

A female CEO, who believes that men don't work as hard as women, questions why women deny themselves opportunity for replenishment. "Is it expectations?" she asks, explaining that many women wouldn't be in their positions if they didn't work harder than men. "This is true even if you've been in your position for a while," she adds. Although she was willing to speak publicly about this, she predicts others won't: "There will be denial about this issue."

Yet some GLHS participants believe the ability to renew themselves is a major strength of women. I did not design the GLHS to yield definitive answers to which sex, if either, is better at the renewal process, but it did produce several noteworthy opinions. One male interviewee reflects the belief of several others in the following comments: "Women are more naturally accommodating of the need to renew, both professional and socially. Women are better positioned to help and build support for each other. They are also more comfortable with admitting their naiveté. Men are more easily 'caught short.'"

One highly placed observer came to acknowledge the importance of practicing personal restoration the hard way—a bout with cancer. That was her turning point, allowing her to "get over being guilty" about taking time for renewing activities more often. Until then, she was like many of her colleagues—"the female health care executives I know don't do much regenerating. They compulsively fill their time," she notes.

Checklist for Renewal

1. As an antidote to the internal drive that pushes you beyond your ability to stop and reflect, ask someone in higher authority to urge or even grant your replenishing opportunities.

2. Find a work environment that supports renewal when you are looking for a new position. Create those opportunities for others who work with and for you—and encourage them to use them.

3. Create opportunities for inspirational activities every day. Without them, and without some free time, transformation can't occur. According to Leland R. Kaiser, "You should allow yourself one hour of free time a day—and it can be filled with any activity, as long as it strengthens you."

4. Obvious, but often neglected: spend time with your family!

5. Dig in the dirt—and don't problem solve or think while doing it. Or run, exercise, keep a journal, read, do whatever it takes to find solace and time for reflection.

6. Find and do the things you like—play music, watch sports, read about science, garden—whatever helps balance your life and your perspective. Doing these things also amplifies your skills.

7. Don't relive the work day. Setting a limit on thinking, processing, or obsessing overtime is a survival skill. It is imperative for renewal.

8. Indulge yourself. Eat chocolate, spend a week in bed, take a year off! Or do all three.

9. Do the unusual. GLHS contributor JoEllen Koerner advises: Take your dishes for a ride!

Section Two: Mentoring Others

Teaching and learning from others is a form of renewal, often called mentoring when it occurs in organizations. As we restore ourselves, nurture our growth as maturing stewards, and groom the next generation of health care leaders, we must rekindle our appreciation for and practice of mentoring. This process is key to continued learning and increased competence, no matter what our stage of leadership. Even for seasoned leaders, mentoring relationships create the opportunity for mutual learning, as well as balanced give-and-take between partners.

Marsha Sinetar, noted expert in personal renewal and prolific author, defines mentoring relationships as those that offer life-affirming spirit. Those who would be mentors embody mature and impersonal love, encouraging us to embrace our authentic selves (Sinetar, 1997). GLHS contributor Myra Isenhart, Ph.D., defines a mentor as an entrusted and experienced counselor or guide and the mentoring process as "learning through relationships."

The traditional mentoring relationship fulfills at least two purposes: career functions and psychosocial functions. Within the former fall classic benefits such as "opening doors," coaching, protection, creating opportunities for visibility, and professional challenge. Within the latter are opportunities for role modeling, counseling, support, and friendship. Mentoring relationships also progress through a series of stages: initiation, cultivation, separation, and redefinition. Initiation and cultivation are the stages most commonly thought of as the mentoring relationship; this is the most active period of teaching and learning (Isenhart, 1996). However, many mentoring relationships continue beyond the most active years, evolving to a meaningful friendship or professional affiliation that both individuals treasure long after the focused initial relationship has subsided.

One GLHS contributor says that, for her, most such relationships have gone from mentoring to friendship, even though they started out as teacher-student relationships: "The period of time for asking for guidance became shorter as I progressed in my career. Now there is more of an interchange."

The Benefits of Mentoring

Research conducted in the late 1980s in business sectors including health care confirmed that individuals who experience extensive mentoring report more promotions and higher incomes. They are also more satisfied with their pay and benefits than individuals who do not experience extensive mentoring. At that time, no gender differences were reported with regard to the frequency of mentoring activities. Also, gender did not moderate the outcome of the relationships (Dreher and Ash, 1990, pp. 539–546).

The Academy of Management found in a 1994 study that women are as likely as men to be mentors in most fields. Among the benefits accrued are the satisfaction and fulfillment received from nurturing the professional and personal development of a protégé. Mentoring can also help improve job performance. But mentoring does not come without its costs, particularly in time and energy. In most organizations, mentoring is not considered part of the job. Also, visibility of the mentoring relationship can magnify both perceived success and failure.

International authority on the Tao Chungliang Al Huang and psychologist Jerry Lynch (1995) offer a view of mentoring that acknowledges these professional and business benefits and embraces the personal benefits as well:

- Mentoring provides an opportunity to slow down, rest, and add to self-knowledge. It reminds us that "we can't see our own image in running water."

- Mentors and mentees receive the ability to learn from and reflect on setbacks.

- Mentors develop loyalty and appreciation of others' growth and professional development.

- Mentors can help to create a safe, nonjudgmental learning environment where all points of view are heard.

- Mentors nurture the ability for others to realize and develop their full potential by confronting and overcoming self-doubt and fear, which is especially important for women.

- Mentors help to ignite enthusiasm and passion in their protégés, as well as to reignite it in themselves.

- Mentoring affords its participants the ability to change places—to serve as an expert in one context and a student in another.

Study contributor Kathryn E. Johnson observes that people will take more risks when they have support in a mentor relationship. This may be particularly true during turbulent times, when there is a heightened need for continuity in learning alliances.

Who Makes a Good Mentor?

We tend to think of mentors as our "superiors" or experts in their chosen fields and our own, and often mentors are just that, modeling the behaviors, traditions, characteristics, and skills we need to learn. But sometimes mentors are not professional experts at all. GLHS contributor JoEllen Koerner is a highly revered nurse executive who has accomplished a great deal in her local, national, and international communities of practice. During her GLHS interview, she identified her guide as her eighteen-month-old grandson. "He has no ego—and he is fully present," she says. "He has innocence and he is aware of what is possible. He is perfect for what is needed today in health care."

Mentors, however, are not always single individuals. Another accomplished leader of a large national organization says that a forum of peers from around the country plays mentor for her. Although she is the designated head of this group, she deliberately creates opportunities to share leadership and to learn from her colleagues.

Indeed, sometimes mentors aren't even people. Marsha Sinetar, author of The Mentor Spirit, focuses not on the vehicle of the mentor (male, female) but on the core of the experience. This essence or "spirit," according to Sinetar, can come through silence, stillness, a sunset. "From it comes a calling that shows what is possible for you," she says. She cites poet William Butler Yeats who, more than a hundred years ago, expressed a similar sentiment: "Education is not the filling of a bucket, but the lighting of a fire" (Sinetar, 1997).

Despite our familiarity with people as mentors, Sinetar's perspective is important, for it opens possibilities for hearing and learning about our talents and new directions in a wide array of settings. Gene Thin Elk, Native American healer from the Lakota tribe of the Sioux Indians in Wounded Knee, South Dakota, offers relevant comment: "We are related to everything in the universe—we are spiritual beings on a physical journey. We believe more in the unseen world than the seen world, and everything has an inner yearning to be part of the whole. There are two wisdom keepers in the circle of life: the elders and the newcomers" (Thin Elk, 1996).

Mentoring in Health Care

In health care, we know that mentoring relationships can assist in acculturating mentees, according to a survey of 551 medical groups in the United States in early 1993 administered by the Medical Group Management Association (MGMA) (Isenhart, 1996, p. 78). These pairings helped the mentees see the big picture and taught them who to turn to—especially in a large organization.

It was beyond the scope of this study to determine *conclusively* whether mentoring is widely practiced in health care, but this section explores the broad range of anecdotal views reflected in GLHS. As of 1993, 25 percent of the MGMA survey respondents confirmed that they used mentoring as a management development tool. Of these, more than 98 percent said these programs had been very or somewhat successful.

However, most GLHS contributors questioned the frequency of mentoring that occurs either formally or informally in health care organizations today. Their concern points to the need for further research to determine whether and how CEOs and other senior managers are actively grooming women, and men, for top-level positions.

The stakes are high for women and for the organizations that will benefit from their talents. Chapter Two reported the ACHE data of 1990 and 1995, which suggested that women aspire to significantly less than men for their careers. In subsequent chapters GLHS participants have offered many possible explanations for this phenomenon. It is also conceivable that women appear satisfied with lower-level leadership roles because they are not groomed, coached, or encouraged by those in senior positions.

As a developer of leadership education with many national, regional, and local organizations for the past twenty years, I have regularly interacted with committed, well-intentioned health care leaders at the highest levels. Yet despite all my positive experiences, and they have been many, I am still left with concern about our willingness to make good on our frequently voiced belief in mentoring. Despite the constant call for grooming up-and-coming leaders with adequate preparation at all levels, most health care organizations still focus much of their attention and educational resources on today's senior leaders. In each instance the decisions may be efficacious, but the result is a paucity of *leadership grooming*—not mere *skill building*—options for potential leaders.

Attesting to the importance of this need, some GLHS participants identified specific benefits of mentoring they received early in their careers. For example, Lillee Gelinas, senior nurse executive with the 1,400-hospital-member VHA, Inc., says she had significant mentors and mentor relationships, including those from her graduate program at the University of Pennsylvania. "There was considerable social learning, in addition to classroom learning," she says.

Others were also thoughtful about their beliefs about and roles as mentors. A fifty-five-year-old CEO of a very large concern examines her mentoring practices, questioning if she is doing a good job of them. "Younger women are so bright—so much more so than I was at their age," she says. "Yet, I have the sense that they are not fully developed as humans. Perhaps it is because many of them were educated with men in MHA programs. I know they had a tough time, but maybe, because of that, they find it easier to deal with men. I wish I understood this better."

Hudson Birden, the health officer for New Britain, Connecticut, noting that mentoring is not always a smooth road, poses an important question: "Should we model ourselves after another, or should we be ourselves? To me, mentoring means that the mentee learns everything the mentor knows, and then goes beyond the mentor. At a broader level, we apply strategies we see others using—

this is learning behavior." In other words, we can do both—use others as role models while refining our own talents and skills.

The voices of the GLHS focus group of twenty-eight to thirty-five-year-olds were strong and uniform in their views of mentoring. These eight individuals all have at least master's degrees in health care management, and several are physicians, nurses, and attorneys as well. Each holds a responsible position in a major health care concern, but not at a senior level. Significantly, none of them has a mentor. Their ardent comments made it clear they see a void for their generation. They believe that the men and women in positions of power and leadership are "Too busy to mentor us, they don't understand us, and they don't take the time to understand where we are coming from."

Mentoring for Women (and Men)

For women, the role of mentoring is an ancient one, rooted deep in Greek mythology and the actions of Athena, the goddess of wisdom and war. Mentor was a friend of Odysseus, who, on departing for Troy, confided to him the care of his house and the education of his son, Telemachus. His name became a proverbial one for a wise and faithful advisor or monitor. Leaving Mt. Olympus, Athena assumed Mentor's shape to help Odysseus in Troy and to help Telemachus find his long-absent father. We can thank her for aiding men and women in their quests for answers.

Trying to sort out the value of same-sex and mixed-sex mentor relationships masks a more basic truth: that men and women each have much to teach the other in all aspects of leadership—and so it is with mentoring. GLHS contributor Eunice Azzani captures the essence of this lesson: "If we truly want to transform our health care organizations, women must mentor men and vice versa. Cross-pollination must occur." Study contributor Cathy Michaels adds that "mentoring is a process in which mutual value is placed on all beings, from a man on the street to a cat. It is leadership and it is followership."

A male contributor's comments echo those of two executive recruiters: that most successful women in health care have had mentors, and mentoring is more important than ever. "The pathways to leadership are very restricted," says Dennis Pointer, Ph.D., who is active at the board level in a number of national concerns. "There is a very strong 'old boys' network, and without mentoring, finding top jobs for women is very difficult." He notes that the mentors of most of the successful women he has seen in health care organizations were men, and that mentoring is rarely discussed. Indeed, "Mentorship practice in health care is invisible," he adds.

Some women do not experience mentoring, or if they do, they do not receive it from another woman. GLHS contributor Roxane Spitzer says that she had only one female mentor—all the others were men. Now at the peak of her leadership career, she is committed to developing other women. For Spitzer, mentoring is about more than education. "It is also about listening, making mistakes, learning from them, and accepting them," she says. Contributor Heidi Boerstler, J.D., is adamant that mentoring, particularly for women aspiring to top leadership roles, is "absolutely critical. We must consciously pass this on: 'I believe in myself!'"

Impact of Gender on Mentoring in Health Care

Are women and men as likely to receive mentoring for leadership roles? As cited earlier, women are as likely as men to *be* mentors, but the GLHS and other study data offer conflicting evidence about whether they are equally likely to *receive* mentoring for the most senior posts. According to one credible source, female health care executives do receive substantial mentoring (ACHE, 1996). But of thirty-three female health care executives speaking in a focus group in late 1995, not a single one could identify having "the kind of mentor relationship [with a man or a woman] . . . that would 'take

her under their wing and tell her how to be a CEO someday'"
(Capozzalo, Bisognano, Gaucher, and Ryan, 1995, pp. 1–3).

The GLHS supports these findings; the words of one female participant epitomize the general belief that "women are not mentored—
they find it so difficult they 'give up the trip' to greater leadership
roles."

Are Women Mentoring Women?

One senior health care executive located in the San Francisco Bay
Area describes an attitude among women toward other women of
"let them do it themselves" when it comes to mentoring: "Women
want to make sure 'it' is perfect, and they beat up on themselves if
'it' is not." The "it" this executive refers to may be a woman's perception of herself as mentor, the lessons she may pass on, and the
questions that will surface during the mentor relationship—that
may touch on personal decisions she has not yet resolved.

Ann Morrison and Van Glinow add another perspective to this
phenomenon. Their research with the Center for Creative Leadership in Greensboro, North Carolina, reaffirms that women may face
barriers to advancement greater than men do—and therefore may
need to spend their time advancing their own careers rather than
helping others (Isenhart, 1996). Indeed, GLHS contributor Carla
Wiggins, commenting on the stresses women face in their careers
and personal lives and the limited time they believe they have for
mentoring, observes this very dynamic in health care.

However, some women *are* mentoring other women, according
to several GLHS contributors. One woman, when asked why her
leadership career has been so successful, says she had great mentors,
was very open to learning, and had the ability to ask for help. She
mirrored the beliefs of Huang and Lynch in her interpretation of
the mentor relationship: "The mentor has a gift; this [fills] a void in
another; it works through that person, and is returned to them both.

This same woman, also a mentor for another woman, identified
some pitfalls of holding such an influential position in guiding the

leadership development of another: "The mentor does not always have good news. In this case, it's important to balance what one says about areas for improvement with strengths. It is also important to consider timing, show respect for the individual, have compassion, and point out things they do well so that they can hear and value your opinion."

Are Women Mentoring Men?

Few male GLHS contributors had female mentors, but two participants did—in fact they had several. William G. Gonzalez, president and CEO of Butterworth Health System in Grand Rapids, Michigan, describes his experience: "My first female mentor was a true mentor. I was impressed by her . . . and her willingness to teach me—she would go to any end to answer my questions. I never felt she was given true credit—or she probably would have been the top finance officer much earlier."

Another man described two of his mentors. Of one, he says, "She had many good qualities, she was a good listener, and she could confront and make hard decisions." From the other, he learned how not to do things. "She was reactive—I learned that you don't put things in writing when you are angry," he says. "They nailed her with a lawsuit!"

Expectations of Mentors

Studies of women mentoring women report that they sometimes discover such relationships to be unsatisfying. Senior women, for example, can feel either discounted or overburdened. Unresolved or unconscious family issues also enter into these mentoring relationships, as we see in these scenarios:

- *My Mentor, My Mother.* Early family experiences can be unconsciously carried into the relationship. The junior member (mentee) may find the relationship repelling rather than compelling. The senior member can also be apprehensive—will the protégé expect perfection?

- *The Search for Self*. Many senior women have already made difficult choices regarding their identity. Perhaps they made choices different from those the protégé would make. Will the protégé then not identify with the mentor? Perhaps the protégé finds the senior woman's confidence daunting.

- *The Search for the "Perfect" Mentor*. Do protégés expect too much? Sometimes they complain when the mentor is hurried and unavailable. Also, senior women may have had male mentors and use that masculine model, perhaps overemphasizing career-oriented functions rather than psychosocial functions such as counseling and friendship.

- *Women Go No Further*. There is a tacit assumption on the part of some females that male mentors are better able to sponsor and promote them. Until now, this has had some basis in fact—the males have been in the senior positions that would afford those opportunities (Parker and Kram, 1993, pp. 42–51).

In keeping with the gender dynamics discussed in Chapter Four, Parker and Kram offer ways to mitigate these factors. They suggest that female leaders increase their self-awareness; open up the discussion to undermining dynamics; and create a supportive organizational culture for themselves and others.

Barriers to Mentoring—and Ways Around Them

Although barriers to mentoring in health care deserve further study, we can still speculate on reasons they may exist and consider options for change.

The Need to Handle Gender with Care

Though not surprising, some of the most disturbing suggestions of the GLHS came from men who voiced concern about mentoring women. Several stated that men simply "have to be careful," as they believe the mentor-mentee relationship can easily be misunderstood either by those outside it or in it. One man who would like to mentor says he thinks about the potential negative consequences of mentoring women "all the time." Still another says "It is difficult for males to mentor females, and it is more difficult now, as an artifact of a litigious environment." He added that a spouse's self-confidence and self-development are key in how close a male can be to a female mentee.

Another participant spoke of internal barriers when mentoring women, explaining that he has more affinity with men, as they remind him of himself. Because he recognizes this tendency, he says "I go out of my way to consciously mentor women." He also acknowledged the possibility of perceived sexual overtones: "I also do not put women in what could be compromising positions—for example, going on a consulting trip. I will not invite them, if they or I will be compromised."

Women, too, express concern about the male-to-female mentoring mix. One woman, about fifty, talks about how difficult it was, even in a supportive environment, for her as a young woman with a male mentor: "There is often a paternalistic flavor or nature to the mentoring. The tension is tough, particularly for younger women. It's hard to separate—they ask themselves, 'Why is this man interested?'" She continues, "How can men and women separate what they are when they are relaxing?"

In these circumstances, men and women are well advised to pursue mentoring relationships that are not also fraught with anxiety about unwanted sexual involvement, or the perception of such involvement. A man working with a gifted woman might arrange for her to work more closely with another successful woman, or with a man for whom entanglement will not be an issue. Women should take the initiative to seek advice and a mentoring relationship with a woman or man they admire whenever the reality or appearance of compromise on the relationship's purpose is not an issue. In either case, both potential mentor and mentee will do well to craft, and recraft over time, the relationship without compromising the professional standing of the other.

Creating Mentoring Options in Large, Hierarchical Organizations

Mentoring relationships can thrive when the participants are stationed within different strata in large organizations. Ideally, opportunities exist to interact professionally and socially. Yet strictly hierarchical institutions may not provide a conducive atmosphere for mentoring if they too closely guard information, privilege, and rank. With care, however, such organizations in health care can successfully put mentoring and learning programs into place, as has been done by complex, large organizations in other industries.

. . . .

A Mentoring Success Story

Myra Isenhart, a specialist in organizational development in the Rocky Mountain Region who focuses on mediation and conflict management, was consulting in the mid–1990s for Kaiser Permanente. In the process, one doctor said that he wanted to take advantage of the clinical skills and leadership potential of women doctors entering the system. As an organizational development expert, she became involved in developing a solution.

"Within a year, I was doing my leadership development work with twelve female physicians, and they initiated three programs. Several years later, two of those three—a colloquium and the mentoring program, which the men also wanted—are still going. Mentoring and networking were identified as the two most prominent needs. Finding time to meet with the female physician managers was difficult, but soon we were off and running with two-hour quarterly meetings. We continue to hear speakers, network with community and women leaders in medicine, and we react to organizational policy.

"The male executives love the mentoring program! Why? Because no one else ever thanks them! It is such a plus to have one relationship in which this occurs. The physician mentors have a chance to pass on their experience as problem solvers. The mentees benefit from advice and career development.

"The women in this experience were really inspiring. None of them went into medicine with the idea that they would be administrators. Management is often not considered 'real work' in the sense that medicine is, and they are not doing it for the 'pitiful pittance' they receive for the big-time headaches of medical management. They want to see things work better. The Kaiser mentoring program is now one of equal opportunity—it's there for men too!"

Taking Time to Mentor

A GLHS participant and keen health care observer comments on the ever-present problem of having too much to do and too little time to do it: "People are so busy that there is little mentoring. [For those trying to learn] it becomes a matter of simply 'watching' people you believe are successful. For people who are beyond school, even this practice drops off, and the situation worsens." He adds, "Then, it becomes a 'dog-eat-dog' world. People are too busy—and we become a closed industry. Therefore, we lose a lot of what we could learn."

We will do well to accept that being a mentor or a mentee is necessary for professional growth. Its value more than makes up for any time spent. Mentoring does not always mean face-to-face interactions. Phone calls, computer conferencing, and even simple e-mails are also effective ways to communicate between one-on-one meetings.

Finding the Resources to Support Mentoring

Until recently, one well-known large organization sponsored a successful mentoring program. But according to one of the study's participating senior nursing leaders, "It went away when we were clamping down." This familiar litany comes from health care concerns that ratchet down financial support for education as a short-term cost-cutting action, believing the program will soon be brought back. But usually these decisions aren't turned around—at least not in the short run. Such expedient choices are anything but wise for those organizations that stand by the need to nurture their current leaders and develop their new ones.

Summing Up

This chapter concludes Part Two by considering the benefits and options for personal renewal and mentoring and their relationships to female leaders. There is uniform agreement among the GLHS interviewees that the need for both approaches is vital for leadership excellence.

We introduce Part Three with Chapter Nine, which focuses on transformation and authenticity. It discusses gender as it relates to leadership, aging, and stages of maturity, and it examines the essence of authenticity for both men and women.

Part III

. . . .

Embracing Authenticity and Power

9

Gender's Role in Transformation and Authenticity

G ender's impact isn't the same as it used to be, say many GLHS contributors. This chapter considers the role of gender as men and women evolve to roles of greater influence, and GLHS con-clusions about gender's impact as these leaders age. It contemplates these questions from a broader social perspective, as well, examining the stages of mastery and wisdom many individuals pass through as they mature.

Finally, this chapter considers transformation in its full measure, extracting qualities, costs, strategies, and tips for achieving authen-tic leadership over the course of a day and over the course of a career. Authenticity here is defined as essence—who we are at our core once we become fully integrated human beings.

To begin, we consider GLHS participants' views about gender's influence on their practice of stewardship over time. Most corre-spondents say the role of gender changes as we mature.

The Male View

Several men who answered the question about the role gender has played as they have evolved commented on gender prejudice. Two believe they have overcome the biases of their upbringings, and in doing so have become more liberated. Several other men attribute change to more indirect processes, such as developing greater comfort with ambiguity. One says that he is more frequently able to move out of his traditional role as a male who "knows the answers," and another is more comfortable saying if and when he has made a mistake.

Gail Sheehy reports these same perspectives in her 1995 book *New Passages,* in which she describes the cycle she terms the "sexual diamond." For the first ten years of life, males and females are very much alike; at puberty, the sexes diverge dramatically; they reach the greatest differences in their late thirties. In their fifties, the sides of the diamond begin to converge again, becoming more like one another in about the mid-fifties. Then, males tend to take on female attributes and vice versa. "Injunctions about what it is to be a man or woman lose force as we age," she writes. "Rigid role divisions melt away" (Sheehy, 1995, p. 318).

The Female View

Many more females elected to answer the survey query about the role gender plays as they age. By far the largest number of respondents, at least a dozen, remarked that they are growing more comfortable with themselves as they mature. A compilation of their stikingly consistent comments illuminates how women leaders settle into themselves as they grow older:

Feminine Style Becomes More Comfortable. Although uncomfortable with their femininity in their earlier leadership years, several contributors say that with age comes comfort. They report receiving more support for their styles and more comfort with their own assessments of other people's character. Several say they are no longer oriented to power and the traditional positional approach to executive practice—now they have greater trust in what one called "group think" and interpersonal relationships.

Lack of Perfection Does Not Limit Power. One CEO says she has "learned to live with the warts and pimples—both my own and those of other people." Several others say they feel more confident and believe more in their own power, even as they become more accepting of their personal limitations.

Exhibiting Some "Male" Characteristics Is Acceptable. At least two GLHS contributors are more willing to display qualities we tradi‐ tionally think of as male. The first, a senior executive in a health plan, says that although process concerned her more when she was younger, "I now have a clearer vision about the end product, while still maintaining the importance of the process." The second, an academic and frequent consultant to health care organizations, says that she is now more comfortable with being direct and clear.

Gender Does Count. Two participants are more willing to acknowl‐ edge gender as a factor in their leadership interactions. "I am now more vocal about gender issues," says a chief nursing officer. "I also use it generously in my interactions. Men don't hesitate to use what they have—why should I?" Another woman, an executive recruiter, comments that she has "become more frustrated with the glass ceil‐ ing. I don't remember being this frustrated earlier in my career."

Willingness to Draw on Both Sides. GLHS interviewee Gates McKibbin, Ph.D., a consultant to major organizations throughout the country, draws on both male and female qualities. From the "male" perspective, she analyzes the competitive environment, industry shifts, and the like. "Knowing war-based metaphors is a critical component to organizational success," she says, but adds that the female viewpoints of the social system and how to support peo‐ ple in their efforts are equally important. "Finding the common ground is key," she says.

Moving Beyond Gender. Two contributors say they have learned to reach beyond their gender socialization, and each noted that she doesn't have to "act like a man" to be successful. These are pivotal insights, and we will return to them later in this chapter and in Chapter Ten.

Examining Our Stages of Wisdom

Sheehy and others provide sociological context for the GLHS lead‐ ers' perceptions of gender's role. Sheehy describes a growing sense of mastery among women, and observes also that women are finding considerable "excitement" in being with other women in the work-place and elsewhere (Sheehy, 1995, pp. 229–235). I have observed this in my own executive-development career. What arises in women of strong vision coupled with the seasoning of experience is a profound passion for new solutions in health care practice. These dreams are nurtured with courage and even bravado and encompass many levels of concerns about health—from new models of well-being and bedside care, to new approaches to leadership through mutual discovery, to new attention to language.

Whereas many women in their late forties and fifties experience a resurgence of energy and commitment, men may find this time of life a much harder transition. This can be particularly true for white males, as we saw in Chapter Seven. Not only have they had the better jobs that women now seek, but they have also been the greater authorities in their families. Sometimes this passage brings with it the unwanted call for men to give up being the "master." Indeed, men may feel "stale, restless, and unappreciated at the precipice of midlife. Often their achievements have left little room for their other emotional and spiritual needs" (Sheehy, 1995).

Women, however, are actively creating new persona and reaching for mastery in new ways. GLHS contributors' statements about increasing clarity and intellectual prowess are confirmed by the findings of sociological researcher Ravenna Helson. For more than twenty-five years, Helson followed 101 female graduates of Mills College, Oakland, California, ages twenty-two to fifty-two. Although these women came from relatively well-to-do homes and had received a good education, they were more dependent, insecure, and self-critical in their younger adult years than their male counterparts. Once they reached fifty and beyond, however, they developed more self-confidence (Sheehy, 1995, p. 194).

Nearly 60 percent of the GLHS interviewees were between the ages of forty-five and fifty-five. At least eight of the women disclosed that they were undergoing profound changes of course in their careers. These women are not being pushed out through mergers or restructuring. Nor are they "dropping out" as a result of a mid-career crisis. Rather, they are making sometimes difficult choices to redirect their energies to fulfill new visions, which are decidedly greater than their previous dreams. Indeed, these women are taking hold of the reins on their careers as never before. They are engaging in risky new ventures, and they are speaking up—and being heard— as acknowledged experts. They are commanding considerable amounts of money for projects that will benefit their communities' health and attracting many other professional women and men who want to join their creative ventures. Singly and together, they are impressive.

What is this metamorphosis? Are these women being edged out of their old existence and into new ones because our organizations cannot accommodate their vision? Is this a crisis of meaning, or a coming of age? The distinct excitement of these women during the interviews strongly suggests the latter. We can conclude they are on the road to what Joan Borysenko describes in her work A Woman's Book of Life (1996): "Through our growing awareness and power, women . . . are helping to birth a new world."

From Survival to Mastery

In his research on career development among professionals, Levinson concludes there is evidence to document these profound transitions for some women, who in their younger career years "are more likely to compromise and put up with situations that are undesirable" (Borysenko, 1996, p. 156). GLHS contributors suggest other ways to look at this phenomenon, which are most succinctly summed up by author and naturopathic physician Farida Sharon. In writing about women's natural receptivity, she states: "For the first 35 to 40 years, we [women] take the world into our being. Many women reach a saturation point around menopause where we cannot take in any more. We have to clear. We have to empty. We have to find our essence again" (Borysenko, 1996, p. 155).

Whatever the case, women reach a state of comfort, ease, and confidence as they mature. When coupled with their increasing focus, clarity, and intellectual prowess, they can become powerful forces for change, and their impact is all the more potent when they are working with men. (Chapter Ten focuses on just such mastery.)

The Transformation to Authenticity

Women and men leading change in health care exhibit the ability, described well by a Hindu proverb, to transform themselves: "The true nobility is to be superior to your previous self." As these men and women move from one stage of leadership to another, they undergo a personal and social journey, which may include a struggle to overcome accumulated baggage, so that they may finally operate with greater ease and authenticity.

Authentic presence, in Tibetan tradition, literally means "field of power." Cooper and Sawaf (1997) tell us what happens when we are in this state: "When we live from 'authentic presence,' from the inside, we can talk openly and honestly with each other, and say the things we deeply feel, even when it's hard to say them. We hold ourselves, and each other, accountable to our best effort in all things. We search for our calling, for the path we are born to take. Every person has this, and can face hardships and problems but not let them live inside them" (p. xxi). This is the search for meaning that "isn't out there, it's in here." From this essence, our spirits can communicate, according to Gene Thin Elk (1996), the healer from the Lakota Nation: "This will help us return to our hearts and our spirits" in the healing professions.

Authenticity, then, is the point at which being and doing are integrated. From here, action flows from values, and we no longer feel the need to make *all* things right. At this point, others who are in the same space will resonate with us naturally. We are reminded of the ancient Chinese philosopher Lao Tzu, who hundreds of years ago stated simply, "The way to do is to be."

Leland R. Kaiser, Ph.D., talks persuasively about this state of being. "People tend to take on the properties of the space they occupy," he says, adding, "These spaces include qualities of people, and good spaces . . . can facilitate you. . . . They provide you with a wide opportunity structure—with lots of choices." In a speaking engagement, Sheila Ryan, dean of the School of Nursing at the University of Rochester Medical Center, counseled (1996) that the quest for authenticity is nurtured in environments without denial. In these places, we can reexperience original wisdom and be true to ourselves *in the world.*

Kaiser goes on to talk about the importance of finding these spaces so we can become our true and authentic beings: "Most people live in one room of their 'house.' Transformation isn't comfortable inherently—there's a loss of security. But if we play it safe, we can't transform."

Many GLHS contributors describe a very clear sense of their movement toward authenticity. Among seven open-ended choices that included topics covered earlier such as communication, conflict management, renewal, and mentoring, at least a third of the contributors chose to comment on "leading with authenticity." One nurse executive tells this poignant story about reaching this expressive and freeing stage of her leadership. You will understand her request that I withhold her name.

> For years the Chief Financial Officer (CFO) in my organization had denied me important financial data and had just cut a large number of staff RNs. I was very concerned about the effect this would have on caring for patients. I decided that this was the 'hill to die on' and I prepared myself to confront him in a meeting with all the senior managers—all males—the next day. But neither he nor the CEO was there. I said to the group that I had wanted to 'call the question' at this meeting—that up until now the staff reduction process was not serving patients or the

organization—but since neither the CEO nor CFO was present, I would not offer my concerns. The other team members encouraged me to speak anyway.

So I did. I told them I had had a dream the night before. *There was a pile of steaming manure in a large field. I pulled out a knife from the pile, and without cleaning it, I castrated the CFO. He had to go to the Intensive Care Unit, but there were only a few nurses left—not enough to take care of him—but there were no others available.* Sharing this story led to the best conversation this group had had in years. But I was very ashamed, and I apologized to each man there. Each one volunteered that he was not going to pass on this story to the CFO.

Although I was intent on the message, I felt very badly about expressing it at this man's expense. To this day, no one has told him this secret. I am not proud of this story. It took me several years to forgive myself for doing this.

This contributor's story vividly communicates the power of standing up with conviction and relaying a message that must be stated, even at the cost of personal discomfort. Most telling is the respect that this contributor had within this group of her peers—all males—who choose to honor the CFO and her by keeping this discussion to themselves. Most important: the outcome was that, after a subsequent group discussion, resources available for acute patient care were increased and ongoing financial data were provided.

The Face of Authenticity

Study contributors offer personal accounts about the forms authenticity can take while leading and collaborating at the executive table:

Authenticity Is Honesty. For GLHS contributor Cathy Michaels, Ph.D., R.N., leading with authenticity "is very key. I feel like pulling back when something doesn't ring true for me."

Authenticity Is Credibility. Authenticity for physician and GLHS contributor Joel Shalowitz means credibility, citing the example of physician leaders. "To be credible, especially with your peers, physician administrators need to know more," he says. "A leader is not only a colleague; he should be a role model. Leaders as 'experts' are part of the same phenomenon, and this has an impact on credibility. In clinical settings, credibility comes from practicing *today*, even if you have already been practicing for forty years."

Authenticity Is Generating Trust. GLHS interviewee Sharon Lee, R.N., M.B.A., believes, "If you are not authentic, people see through you and you will lose effectiveness as a leader. Trust is critical." Another CEO says about trust, "If I can't give all the information, I say so up front. [Trust] means having good interpersonal skills; it means trying not to lie; it means admitting mistakes when you've screwed up, and asking for help or support when you need it."

Authenticity Is Leading from Values. GLHS contributor Roxane Spitzer, Ph.D., R.N., says, "We bring our basic values into leadership, and they strengthen and develop over time. Values are critical to being an effective leader of any kind." She believes that character is learned, that it means "trust, integrity, risk taking, vision, engendering real support from staff, and communication skills—listening and hearing, not just talking."

Authenticity Is Assumed. People assume that you are authentic until you prove otherwise, says Pam Thompson, R.N. And they know it when the leader proves otherwise. A high-ranking public health official talks about a colleague with a "big knowledge deficit. Everybody knew this. He further compounded the problem by surrounding himself with people less competent than himself. He created an inept administration, and he was in office for several years as evidence was gathered to support what everyone instinctively knew. Once the data was in, he was canned."

Authenticity Is True Caring. For GLHS contributor Jennifer Kosakowski, caring is 99 percent of authenticity: "Authentic people are not necessarily admired, but their circle of concern is much bigger than just themselves. . . . Its presence builds loyalty."

Authenticity Is Honoring Your Heritage. Kathy Reno, a successful nurse executive in a large urban hospital, recounts her experience of coming to terms with authenticity. This involved publicly acknowledging she had come from what she labeled a fairly poor background. "We didn't consider ourselves poor, but it was hard to talk about this for the first ten years of my career," she says. "But, when I let this become part of who I am, I became more comfortable and then could engage with staff nurses. . . . I make fun of myself with them—for example, saying I read romance novels." The number one factor in success is being who you are, she counsels, adding, "You don't have to think, plot, or whatever. You don't have time to do this anyway."

Authenticity Is Being the Same—Regardless of the Setting. One GLHS interviewee reports that no matter where he is, he doesn't change: "My challenges are the same in my personal and professional lives. My actions are consistent with my values."

Authenticity Is Stepping Aside—For a Time. A sixty-year-old CEO whose company was merging with a much smaller institution in the area offers his view of being authentic. "The other institution fears consumption by this system," he says. "Miraculously, we have been given an opportunity in which the other guy will be CEO for the first year and a half—and after that I will be CEO. I sense that this way, the merger will have a chance of working."

Authenticity Is Power. Power relates to authenticity and self-renewal, believes GLHS contributor Gates McKibbin, Ph.D. "My deepest power comes from inner work, and it comes from light and shadow," she says. "Recognizing both, I have less to hide, deny, run away from—this helps me be more authentic. Therefore I embrace my power. Ultimately, I believe power comes from courage and authenticity—the strength of the heart is the act of the sword."

Authenticity Is Moving Beyond Gender. According to GLHS contributor Linda Burnes Bolton, Ph.D., R.N., "Gender makes less difference now as we are authentic, real, and visible. People will see if you are real. This will be true no matter what position you are in.

Come forward with what you can do, say you can do it, and then really do it! It's okay to say 'I am able to do X, I need help with Y, and I know where to get it.' Check the ego, and demonstrate what you can accomplish."

Authenticity Is Reflection. A significant tool in the transformation to authenticity is reflection. GLHS contributor JoEllen Koerner, Ph.D., R.N., writes (1996) that reflection facilitates learning through practice—an essential and core element of professional competence. Koerner and others have observed the artifacts of professional socialization we examined in Chapter Two, noting that such indoctrination can create barriers "because the focus is on technical rationality versus reflection-in-action."

Koerner is a remarkable health care leader in *many* respects, contributing her wisdom and vision to growing communities of healing throughout the United States, Australia, and New Zealand. She described to me her path toward gender and spiritual integration as she has matured into her fifties. She says, "Coming from a Mennonite background where women were seen and not heard, I have gone through many stages—the passive good girl, the furious feminist, the pleaser, pleader, the pragmatic. Today, I am free to make choices that go beyond emotion." She sees gender as one of many variables, but not one that controls or drives her. She also feels she has great affection and compassion for difficult people, but is grateful she can say "go to hell" if necessary. She adds, "I look at my twenty-eight-year-old daughter and realize that it is terribly important to share this perspective. For me, this is a quantum leap forward in being human."

GLHS interiewee Jane Neubauer believes that "finding space to reflect, think, get support, and get to know oneself better is critical." She says she didn't have that space during her executive career in the early years. Although she frequently traveled to meetings, she mostly just had a short break, did a bit of networking, and complained. "Being authentic doesn't just happen—you need space to explore who you are," she says. "As more opportunity for reflection evolves, there is the potential for people to be less stressed if they can be more authentic at work. Maybe this will entice women to stay in organizations." She speculates that men may be less likely to access this type of development initially, but once they are involved, they will recognize the same need for reflection and balance in their life.

Painful but Productive

One GLHS contributor now in her early forties hopes her story will encourage others. "In the early 1990s, my boss told me I would not become a partner in the firm," she says, pointing out that usually when women get these messages, they work harder and their supervisors take advantage of this. "I worked really hard, too—in fact, I only took off two weeks to have my third child. Subsequently, three women made the criteria for partner. None was promoted.

"I took this, and the fact that I was consistently underpaid, to an excellent attorney, who said this was a clear-cut case of discrimination, but that the remedy would be partnership. This firm had been sued many times. I decided that becoming a partner in that firm was not worth it, and that I was going to leave. I did so, and told the firm that I wouldn't settle for anything less than a female-friendly environment.

"I put myself in the driver's seat as I looked for a new job. I knew I would take only a partnership. All I had to do was deliver, which I knew I could do. I looked for indicators about the environment, I met with senior people one on one, and held conversations that would go deep into issues. I would 'test' them, and not just on the 'female' issue. I asked: 'How old are the people? No matter what their ages, are they cutting the trail?' Some firms dropped out, as they didn't like the hurdles I erected. I established my style on the front end—I was open and direct."

This contributor landed a highly prized partnership in a new firm and has done very well for the clients, the firm, and herself in the years since.

In sum, these leaders define authenticity as a way of being that leads to operating credibly and honestly based on values. For some, it is honoring one's personal or professional heritage or electing to take lesser leadership roles. All of the GLHS participants embrace transformation and evolve to a new stage of authenticity when they do the following:

- Engage in self-examination and reflection

- Understand their true internal values and use them to guide their choices of professional commitment

- Communicate honestly about their views and their goals, as well as about the skills they may not possess

- Make choices that go beyond emotion and act on them

The Price of Authenticity

The courage these individuals demonstrate comes with a price— and sometimes it is steep. GLHS contributor Phyllis Kritek sees it this way: "People who think you have to pay with your soul are served notice by authenticity in others. Authenticity can be viewed as attacking, stepping out of role, being disturbed, being disturbing, and a variety of even stronger words. The system says authenticity means 'breaking the rules.' Authenticity is hard to come by, and it is rarely rewarded." Kritek is known and acknowledged for her work with conflict and negotiation in nursing. Of herself in this regard she accurately says that she is a credible national figure, but goes on to say that "I am not the norm. I live in a culture that does not value truth, that instead wants recipes. How do you have wisdom in a culture that only values knowledge?" She says that people do forgive a lot if intentionality is clear and she uses an epitaph—What do I want my life to have meant?—to guide her decisions. For her, rich, famous, and dominating don't do it. She says, "In one way it's the perfect time to be a force for the light, even if we are lonely, and subjected to denigrating messages. We must walk away from costly environments."

The act of walking away may cause conflict, which she relates to authenticity: "Conflict always mirrors that which I have not become, or I have chosen not to become. To be inauthentic evokes being careful and erecting walls with others. Authentic behavior begets different reactions."

The GLHS found at least a dozen male and female health care leaders making the hard choice of genuineness and suffering consequences they were willing to bear. The issues over which they draw the line in favor of authenticity ranged from personal integrity to commitment to quality patient care. At least 50 percent of the women's stories dealt with their unwillingness to accept derisive actions, politics, or comments about females.

Authenticity Means Stepping Out of Role. One female physician describes her recent experience: "I was told '*your role is to do what you are told.*' I said, 'I think you have the wrong person for the job.' I am now managing a medical facility, but I had a higher position before I left. That organization spent six months trying to get me to 'comply' and to keep me."

Authenticity Means Standing Up for Oneself. One GLHS contributor watched her position fall apart five years ago. At XYZ hospital, she developed her job, vice president of patient care services, and the CEO depended on her for credibility with the physicians. She was overseeing a $100 million budget and two-thirds of the organization reported to her. Then a new CEO arrived. "He spent the first year chipping away at my power and authority with the clinical staff," she recounts. "The CFO didn't want to give me so much power either, because the organization was financially distressed. The quality of patient care was terrible—it should have been the first thing we attended to. But instead, they diminished my role, hiring another woman with no operational experience to replace me. I stood up for myself, and left. It was very hard for me, but I left knowing I had stood by my principles and that I would land on my feet." She did!

Authenticity Means Asking for, then Demanding Respect. Still another woman described her experience working in a highly responsible health care position in city government in a sophisticated urban area in the early 1980s. In her early thirties at the time, she was the only woman on the executive staff. One of the staff members repeatedly made comments about "the girls," and a member of the city's Board of Supervisors called women "the dollies"— or worse. She was told to do the health briefings for this individual but, concerned about harassment, she refused. "I had the intellect, and their respect," she says. "They knew I would leave if they did not honor my wish. It was early enough in my career and my husband and I were not locked into our location. I felt I could take such a risk." They honored her wish.

Choosing Your Battles

Some leaders will not choose the path of authenticity, at least not every time. One study contributor comments on an essential dilemma common to some other contributors: if a leader is not immediately concerned with survival on the job, impact is often the goal. "Authenticity isn't always the shortest distance between A and B," she says. "One may have to deviate from authenticity to exercise power." Another described her experiences as a partner at a consulting firm early in the 1990s. One partner left, and a client said he would not deal with a "different" partner—in other words, with a woman. "We either had to reassign the client or let him go as a customer," she says. "As a woman, I was told not to even make a presentation to this client."

But soon after, another client helped to change the policy at her firm. The COO of a major customer account demanded female presence on the consulting team. "If the client had not done this, there would be no incentive for my firm to change," she says. "Frankly, it was easier to fight City Hall. This was a game that could not have been won without that client's insistence, and for me as a woman, it was not a hill to die on."

The Hero at Work

Through these heartfelt tales, we begin to appreciate that the quest to and through authenticity can take the health care leader to a form of modern-day heroism. We think of heroes as endowed with great strength or ability, achievement, courage, and admirable qualities. Prolific author Joseph Campbell's definition of a hero (1997) fits best with the transformational leadership path: "The essence of a hero is the ability to live from the heart and to be human."

One GLHS contributor, operating at the highest level of a large national institution, defines heroism as staying on the job in the midst of the sea changes that have occurred in the health care system during her tenure. "After nearly thirty years, I am still in the same organization. My personal success is based on partnership and collaboration. I put those before my own personal gain."

Mark Strand, former Poet Laureate of the United States, eloquently describes where such genuineness and focus can take a leader: "You're right in the work, you lose your sense of time, you're completely enraptured, you're completely caught up in what you are doing. When you are working on something and you are working well, you have the feeling that there's no other way of saying what you're saying" (Csikszentmihalyi, 1990, p. 62).

We know these moments best by experiencing them. For Sandra Hernandez, M.D., these qualities lead to personal service, which for her is the *raison d'etre* of health care leadership. In a recent speaking engagement, she expressed her concern that health care has "shifted from personal service to cost containment." She is not alone in this concern, nor in her allusion to leadership's purpose. Emmett Murphy, author of *Leadership IQ* (1996), surveyed thousands of successful leaders in a number of industries, including health care. His findings show that benchmarked leaders do *everything* on behalf of the customer.

Summing Up

This chapter focuses on the role of gender as men and women move into greater leadership roles, and the stages of mastery and wisdom they pass through as they mature. It considers the qualities and consequences of making the choice for authenticity. Seven simple tips are the gist of living authentically every day:

Be able to live with yourself. Elaine Cohen, Ph.D., acknowledges that leading authentically is very difficult: "I need to look in the mirror—literally—and like what I see. If I can't do that, then I'm working in the wrong place. I learned this from a powerful mentor, and it is not easy to do."

Work with passion. Carol Spain, M.P.H., advises "picking something you feel passion for—then you can be real about it. If you invest yourself, your passion, and your creativity, the result will be meaningful. . . . But when you are not clear and decisive, allow yourself to be a little vulnerable. Doing this allows others to . . . know that you are open to their ideas and perspectives."

Check your ego at the door. For Nando Zepeda, M.P.H., "It is easier to function when you understand your own ego needs—you are better able to be in service to others. There is not a real leadership 'style' or ready-made tools. Bring yourself and the behavior that is required. Bring capacities and shape them to what's needed."

Be straight. Distinguished researcher and university dean Deborah Freund describes herself as service oriented and straightforward: "People know they can count on me. I will approach them directly—with problems or whatever. My style is to be direct and brutally honest."

Set up boundaries and stick to them. A highly accomplished CEO who began her career as a nurse says very clearly: "I have never let anyone abuse me. I have always known who I was and I have always been comfortable with that. I grew up in a family that was very support-ive and this gave me a lot of self-esteem. You can be what you want to be. In fact, any limitations you have, you place upon yourself."

Know what "hooks" you. "I know that my buttons can be pushed by authority figures—especially male authority figures," says one female contributor. "Women can absorb so many feelings, and they can be overwhelmed and paralyzed by them. I've learned to have a thicker skin."

Have courage. One very successful woman in her fifties recounts an experience earlier in her career. She was sitting in a staff meet-ing with the other partners in her firm, and one of the males, who was about fifty-five, said that she would be more successful if "I didn't reveal so much of myself to my clients, and to the world. I told him I was successful *because* I reveal myself. I said if he meant success in terms of business generated, he was accurate. But who was he to say where I would be when I was his age? Perhaps I would be three times more successful than he!" Reflecting on why she did this, she says, "My statement stoked my competitive juices. In every encounter, I learn as much about myself as I do about everyone else. Would I have done this if I were thirty-five? Probably, but I would not have done it in my twenties!"

Chapter Ten integrates the experiences, stories, and wisdom of the GLHS contributors, offering a fresh view of stewardship that encompasses but does not dwell on gender or any other single aspect of leadership excellence. This perspective embraces GLHS con-tributors' beliefs about the most important and enduring qualities of those they admire, coupling them with moving examples of their executive practices on the firing line of everyday life in health care today.

10

. . . .

From Paradox to Power

The stewards of our health face a panoply of challenges, some of them daunting, as we move into the new millennium. Throughout the book, their representatives have led us through their personal experiences and beliefs as they negotiate, face, and sometimes initiate conflict; encourage change and welcome difference; hone skills; renew themselves and their careers; and serve as mentors and mentees.

This chapter explores the state of leadership that underpins the leader's best work. It "puts it all together" by looking again at stewardship in health care—this time enabled by the key beliefs and skills described earlier. Through stories of real leadership successes, we glimpse personal and career peaks of achievement. Stewardship at this level acknowledges but is not overcome by gender considerations or barriers. Here, senior leaders convey their message with clarity and mastery.

These inspiring tales mirror the opinions of GLHS contributors' views on two key questions:

1. What are health care leadership's most *enduring* leadership competencies?

2. Are these capacities related to gender, and if so how?

For most study participants, such enduring competencies are simply those required to function optimally on a sustained basis. They may take the form of knowledge and wisdom, expressions of the soul, levels of skill, or products and outcomes.

Their beliefs call for a new term for competencies, one better suited to the most admired characteristics of masterful influence. Renamed "archetypes of leadership," these qualities are ephemeral, take many forms, and are difficult to capture as discrete phenomena. Like archetypes, we simply know them when we see them.

Study contributors offered moving tributes to their colleagues who display these archetypes of leadership, especially when they told stories about one another rather than about themselves.

Gender and Balance in Leadership Archetypes

Respondents' beliefs about gender's relationship to the archetypes are conclusive: gender is *not* a relevant factor in the expression or effectiveness of these traits. A brief summary of their insights reveals these points:

Gender does not determine whether a leader is revered. This conclusion makes sense—once gender is no longer a barrier, whether in ourselves or in how we perceive others, the essential qualities of effectiveness are all that remain.

Lack of awareness about the role of gender in leadership is the issue. When we are unconscious of the impact of gender socialization, health care culture, and our dominant models of leadership, we will evaluate leadership qualities one way. We will respond differently, however, when we are aware of and choose to move beyond the complex intertwining of gender and the other variables that influence leadership life in health care.

Effective stewardship springs from personal integration and gender balance. "Gender is relevant in that all effective leaders work at the intersection of male and female perspectives," says one GLHS contributor. "On the male side, we are in competitive environments with industry shifts and the like," she says. "The other side includes the social systems and structures that are good for supporting people. The key to these perspectives for the effective leader is finding the common ground."

Archetypal Leadership Traits

Archetype One: Wisdom, Knowledge, and Discernment

Being knowledgeable, knowing the limits of that knowledge, and staying abreast of the dynamic environment in which leadership is played out were all listed by more than a dozen contributors as key traits. They revere wisdom, which a top female official eloquently defines: "Wisdom is that which comes from the deepest personal integration of self, while understanding and honoring the other."

Discernment is that aspect of wisdom that enables the leader to balance the masculine and feminine parts of her nature and to be adroit as she uses a full array of skills to accomplish her goals. Because she is prepared, she is able to relax in her work and remain grounded, which enables her to respond appropriately to whatever situation occurs. This archetypal leadership quality takes shape in a leader as she recognizes that she, not her credentials, her beliefs, or any other *part* of her being, is the vehicle for effectiveness. These three stories are testaments to such wisdom:

Her presence is uplifting. A female leader long admired by Hudson Birden, M.P.H., engenders a feeling of calm in those around her because she is never rushed, is always focused, and exudes confidence. The two were on a board of directors whose organization was embroiled in a significant clash with another organization. "As President of 'my' Board," he says, "she stayed focused on our organization's mission, and she did a masterful job of negotiating. She really thought about what was being said, chose her words carefully and did not allow herself to become 'drawn in.' The males around the table, on the other hand, became 'red of face' and 'loud of voice.'"

Balance is a must. Embodying balance is equally important for men and women, says Leanne Kaiser Carlson, M.H.S.A., recalling her earliest role models: "They had a blend of assertiveness and nurturing, collaborative styles. In my experience, it is almost the rule rather than the exception that truly great leaders display this balance, having integrated both the male and female sides of themselves."

Self as vehicle for community benefit. Linda Miller, president and CEO of the Volunteer Trustees of Not-for-Profit Hospitals, named Bettsanne Holmes, member of the board of the New England Healthcare Assembly, as the epitome of a leader with impact. Miller, who works with hundreds of trustees and chief executive officers around the nation each year, paved the way for Holmes to participate in the GLHS.

Although she has encountered her share of gender-related bias, Holmes says this has never stopped her. Strong in her belief that women, who are often the purchasers of health care, know better than anyone how their community regards its health care system, she first came to serve on a health care board as a representative of the women's hospital auxiliary. When she joined the board in this role, she asked the other two women there whether they had a vote. They didn't know. "This was my first problem!" she says.

Eventually Holmes was invited to be a full board member, despite predictions that this would never happen. She then became the first female board chair, despite more predictions to the contrary. Some years later, she agreed to join another board, and asked for a treasurer's report. She was told there wasn't one, that the board had never had one and had operated very well for years without one. "Essentially they said they 'didn't need a young woman telling them how to do their work.' I thought about this—and I decided I'd continue to ask for a report in each quarterly meeting. I did this until they provided one," she says.

"When I am not looked at, not heard, or other people take my ideas, I approach it with lightness," Holmes says. "I am not light in terms of my request for change, information, or whatever, but in terms of my manner. Humor goes a long way, and a little self-deprecation doesn't hurt either."

Holmes never sees herself as a victim. She advises, "If you're put down, refuse to be put down—bounce back up again! When you play their game, play by your rules, don't let them co-opt you. Don't make enemies—be someone they have to deal with."

Archetype Two: Integrity

Character stood out as the most significant enabler of enduring stewardship in the GLHS. Contributors define character in many ways, all of which sum to integrity. Adding to the considerable data that affirm its importance, a study of leadership in the 21st century by Korn/Ferry International (1996) in cooperation with the Economist Intelligence Unit of London, England, cited integrity and the *image* of integrity as key ingredients for powerful leaders. These are leaders who offer no surprises. Confidence and trust can build.

Commonly defined, integrity is the unwavering commitment to moral and ethical principles. But integrity also means "The state of being whole, entire, and undiminished" (Cooper and Sawaf, 1997, p. 174). Integrity, then, is the root of integration—the ability to bring together all parts of ourselves. Contributor Sandra Hernandez, M.D., says integrity is "To answer the same question, the same way, no matter who's asking it." The following three stories embody integrity:

Doing the right thing—even when the price is high. For one physician who requests anonymity, maintaining integrity brought down upon her criminal charges and cost her a prized job. Her mentee tells about this woman, her faculty advisor, who was convicted of manslaughter in her state because she had performed an abortion on a woman who contracted German measles in her first trimester of pregnancy. This illness is associated with extremely severe birth defects. Upon conviction, the advisor had to leave the state. Her student, now a physician, says, "I followed her—learning so much from her. I was able to do important research, perform in-hospital second-trimester abortions for young girls in desperate situations with no one else to help them. Our goal was for women and girls to have a choice."

Shooting straight. Her colleagues praise Jennifer Kozakowski, R.N., M.P.H., for her ability to promote trust. Kozakowski, a managed care expert, attributes that ability to "shooting straight." She gives people constant feedback and creates an environment in which it is okay to learn in "failure." She stresses the importance of recognizing that sometimes eliminating a position, or firing someone, is a kind act. "This gut-wrenching but compassionate confrontation is imperative. I have made a commitment to the employees with whom I work. They know they have signed on for growth and development. Whether I like them is irrelevant. But I do need to care enough about them to guide their work and their careers successfully." And they feel she does.

Shooting straight, no matter what the season. William G. Gonzalez, president and CEO of Butterworth Health System in Michigan, describes a time early in his career when the integrity of a mentoring team member made itself felt: "One year, with a lot of Medicaid changes affecting payments to hospitals, we faced a $3.3 million deficit. As CEO, I was told by the board to 'fix it,'" he recounts. He and his management team concluded in mid-December they would have to lay off about 250 employees, but he couldn't bring himself to tell people before Christmas. So his team decided to wait until after the holiday to notify the staff about layoffs. Several days later, a management team member called "Sumi" told him she could not sleep because of that decision, that she felt horrible. She said, "If you don't announce this to the staff before Christmas, they will spend all their money." She persisted, visiting him three more times, until he finally changed his mind. He announced the layoffs around December 18 or 19 in a series of forums. "During the first one, with more than two hundred people—about 10 percent of the hospital staff—I told them everything, about my initial fear of telling them, about our first decision and about how Sumi had changed my mind.

I said that they needed to know before the holidays and that it would be a greater disservice to them otherwise. When I was done, the whole auditorium stood up and clapped."

Living Integrity as an Archetype

1. Be humble enough for leadership.

2. Don't always assume you are the leader.

3. Know the limits of your knowledge.

4. Don't compromise your values for personal comfort.

5. Be open and available, especially to younger people.

6. Critically evaluate your actions. Check out whether they are generating the trust of others.

7. Make your practice and your philosophy congruent.

8. Live from a base of unconditional love, make positive choices, and be grateful for the opportunity to make a difference.

9. Commit to *absolute* integrity. Former leaders do not get the chance to correct honesty and integrity.

Archetype Three: Key Skills

A leader's competence and skills are among her most significant assets. She must use them wisely in every professional encounter, relying particularly upon a "superskill"—her ability to embrace paradox, ambiguity, and change.

Four practical ways to achieve this superskill get top billing. They are *flexibility*, *self-reflection*, *creativity*, and *assertiveness*.

Flexibility

Flexibility in action is critical. It means the ability to learn quickly and turn around fast—especially from failure. Creating cultures that promote diversity, acknowledge paradox, and embrace difference requires flexibility. Such dexterity becomes an essential ingredient in professional growth for the leader herself, as well as for those with whom she works most closely. As F. Scott Fitzgerald wrote: "The test of a first-rate intelligence is the ability to hold two opposing ideas in mind at the same time and still retain the ability to function."

Flexibility is a transformational skill for success. Connie Burgess had always wanted to own her own business. More than ten years ago she decided to make the leap, an action that permitted her to return to "who she really was." In building her successful managed care consulting practice, she says that she has found it useful to have two business cards. One shows her degrees—M.S., R.N.—the other does not. "If I do not introduce myself as a nurse, I do introduce my knowledge of health care and nursing, but in the context of the discussion," she says. Burgess does this because earlier in her career she was partner with a man not as knowledgeable as she but whom senior health care executives knew better, so they often spoke to him first. "I realized that I had to get their attention, and that I was dealing with several issues—being a woman and being a nurse," she says, adding, "I am tall, and I can cut an imposing picture, particularly when I am 'on.' But I was still experiencing this!" Since then she has "learned their language" and overcome her own trappings: "Most men don't care about the nursing/patient model—they just want the bottom line." This means that she learned to listen better, to stop selling so hard and wait for a well-chosen time to assert her knowledge. "I am comfortable now being direct and straightforward," she says. "When I veer from my own truth, I get into trouble, I feel far less comfortable, and I can become more easily intimidated."

Self-Reflection

The ability to reflect on challenges in quiet and renewing settings is important for leaders who want to be unencumbered by the momentum of escalating reactions. One female contributor begins by asking herself the simple question "How have things gone?"

Doing this allows her to see what compromises can and cannot be made. It keeps her from sacrificing integrity for comfort.

Self-reflection helps maintain vision through adversity. A highly successful CEO of a national health care concern talks about the power of reflection in enacting long-term vision. "During my term as chair of a large national association, I spent a great deal of my time assisting the organization to craft a strategic plan," she says. "The chair following me saw many situations in win/lose terms, and was quite blatantly power-driven. He pushed hard on certain things, and was really appalling in his exercise of power. If things didn't go his way, he'd be gracious but. . . ." Her voice trailed off, then picked up. "During his tenure as chair, he 'forgot' the legacy of my vision—which had been adopted by the organization. This precipitated a moral crisis of sorts for me." On three occasions, she confronted him privately; each time, he acted "shocked." Each discussion was difficult; she chose to direct them by insisting on "finding a way." "Finally, I approached the incoming board chair, a woman. With considerable difficulty and energy expenditure, the situation was resolved positively." Her honesty in assessing her own tactics and how far she would go to maintain the plan stood her in good stead in the end, even as she grew more uncomfortable during the process.

Creativity

For most contributors, creativity means recognizing opportunities, being innovative while using good judgment, practicing detachment, and thinking "outside the box." For others it means having and keeping a sense of humor. This is the ability to reframe situations and the will to take ourselves less seriously.

Creativity is also key to clarifying patterns and encouraging people to learn by playing off each other, sometimes through conflict.

Creativity in contributing to community. Anne Hall Davis has distinguished herself as a health care trustee for many years. As a volunteer community leader, she has long urged health care systems to form planning committees rather than building committees—to stress service rather than bricks and mortar. Acknowledging her contribution to the quality of care in Cape Cod, Massachusetts, she has been asked to serve at the highest levels of governance in the American Hospital Association.

Early on, Davis saw an opportunity through her unique connection to her locale. Unlike most other community business concerns, "My husband's business was *not* dependent on the community for its success, so I could speak for a lot of people because it was not threatening to our survival," she says. "People would feed me their thoughts about their needs. I learned a great deal from many people—and I put it to use in this way." Through her creativity, Davis was primary in starting a psychology service on Cape Cod, then a radiation service, and finally a full-service satellite of Massachusetts General Hospital.

Assertiveness

More than 25 percent of the contributors place assertiveness in league with other enduring skills for leadership excellence. Various interpretations of this trait include holding people accountable, making clear decisions, and taking decisive action. Personal benefits include having the ability and confidence to take risks, being candid and direct, negotiating with "chutzpah," and embodying a drive for success. Courage is also a form of assertiveness, as this story shows:

Asserting boundaries to achieve goals. Barbara Donaho, M.A., R.N., has been assertive at many tables during her long and singularly successful career as nurse executive, senior nursing officer for a major health system, and several-time CEO. Donaho knows who she is and is "comfortable with that." She tells of being offered a two-year contract to assume the chief executive position at a hospital system a few years ago. "But what could I accomplish in two years?" she asked, adding that she told the hospital's negotiating team that if it wanted her, the contract would have to be for five years. The job came through. She offers advice worth repeating: "You can be what you want to be, and any limitations you have, you place on yourself." She urges women to be clear and not to worry that by doing so they won't get the job.

Archetype Four: Getting Results

This archetype represents the tangible outcome of effectiveness, a temporary resting place for achievement, and knowledge that goals have been attained. These may be momentary victories or the achievement of cherished, lifelong pursuits. Results may appear in many forms, including effectively communicating, establishing common ground, or promoting accountability, as these stories describe.

Storytelling. Pam Bromley, former vice president of patient care at St. Alphonsus Health System in Boise, Idaho, reveals one powerful aspect of good communication: the strategic use of storytelling. Bromley's organization wanted to upgrade its helicopter service to remote areas but could not justify doing so on a strictly financial basis—the new equipment would assist only 10 percent of the patients. Yet Bromley knew the purchase would benefit the community. To gain support for the idea, she talked about the patients whose lives are affected by the availability of helicopters. "The hospital was immediately able to see the results in personal terms—family members from remote areas could travel together during an emergency rather than separately, offering the family far greater stability and emotional support," she says. "We got the new helicopter."

Finding common ground. One contributor, a well-respected female with a key position in one of the country's most highly regarded systems, has committed her professional life to creating a common vision of health while enabling the richness of difference. She tells a story of putting this into practice. In the early 1980s, she observed a large number of Filipina nurses in her institution eating together all the time and speaking only their language. Patients were complaining that they didn't understand the nurses, thus adding to their anxiety. When she tried to explain this problem, the Filipina nurses felt she was out to get the them. The other nurses weren't happy either. One nurse manager said to her, "You recruited them, now when they do their jobs, you penalize them."

She was faced with a paradox and a dilemma until she found out that their culture values families highly: "I told a story, saying,

'Imagine your grandfather being frightened.' We talked about how helping families is 'what we are all doing here.'"

Finding the common ground among them set a new course for these nurses—and for her. They compromised, yet still honored their mutual commitment toward family well-being—the nurses could speak their own language as long as they were in private areas. She reflects on her key leadership touchstone: "In situations like this, whatever I do has to pass my litmus test: 'Above all, do no harm,'" she says. "Acknowledge the person first. There may be a struggle, but at least the person gets the message that I am not discriminating."

Accountability and truth. The real heroine of this story is unknown. But a contributing CEO bears witness to her courage, integrity, and singular accountability: "Around 1980 or 1981, a sponge was missing in the operating room. The staff did everything to find it, and concluded that it had been thrown out. But one African-American female was not so sure. She couldn't sleep at night. She went to the surgeon and told him that she had emptied the trash and that the sponge was not there. She also said that she thought she had seen it in a patient's X ray. She retrieved the film and pointed out what she thought was the sponge on the film. She was absolutely correct."

Reflections on the Archetypes

Contributors repeatedly discussed the importance of self-knowledge, the springboard for insight into the ego's needs, allowing us to separate crippling baggage from the tools that will create the best course for health care in the new millennium. Such knowledge enables us to develop our most vital leadership tool: ourselves. It pushes us toward feedback, reflection, and accountability—it lets us show up unfettered for the job at hand. Perhaps most importantly, it allows us to pursue true authenticity by removing the illusion of unfailing personal expertise.

Offering testament to personal accountability among health care leaders, we consider contributor Patrick Hays's 1996 briefing for a national audience of senior health care leaders. After many other candid remarks, Pat paused and stared evenly at his colleagues and friends. He then described, with characteristic sincerity, the enormous arrogance he finds in health care. His comments were brief, yet they had a profound impact on those present. The hushed response was palpable as physicians, nurses, policy makers, and executives considered their part in the truth of his statement.

Through self-mastery, the leader can relinquish such arrogance. Practicing the skills presented in Chapters Five through Nine and considering the examples and qualities of the soul found in this chapter, she can lead without undue concern for gender or other barriers. Instead, she can enter the territory where decisions are made with ease, where discipline and training become natural, and even unconscious, allies. She is beyond the illusory pull of other people, understanding that most people are "neither for you nor against you; they are thinking about themselves" (Gardner, 1996, p. 10).

Here, the health care leader is free to act, to communicate, and to engage the world with clarity. She is free to focus on the task at hand. She can "burn with a clear blue flame."

Burn With A Clear Blue Flame

At this point, the art and craft of leadership come together. Here is where the leader guides with elegance, maturity, and precision. Here, we are in leadership's essence. Here, specific competencies and skills are no longer in focus. Here, our individual features, including gender, fade from undue significance. Here, we experience the expression and impact of true stewardship, whether witnessing it in another or offering it ourselves. Here, distinctions dissolve into wholeness.

We can express leadership without the "stuff" of barriers—the rocks in our packs, the unfamiliar roads that unsettle us, the petty frustrations that make us less than effective, the resentments that we unconsciously communicate to others. We no longer emanate the belief that we are entitled to leadership privilege, even if we are not qualified. We are no longer experts beyond challenge. Here, we live in the present. Here, we *burn with a clear blue flame*.

Contributor and executive recruiter Peter Rabinowitz uses this phrase to describe the essence of women he places in top leadership roles. "Women at this level create safety for others and preserve choices for people, rather than boxing them in. They move beyond personal needs to being comfortable with the personal use of self," he says.

This state of being creates openness, allowing the leader to receive vital information that can come from anywhere within her scope of concern. This feedback allows her intuition—one of mature leadership's greatest assets—to flow in service of the challenge rather than simply her own personal cares. Access to intuition engenders reflection and subsequent right action.

Gender is as relevant at this stage of leadership as any other personal aspects of self, such as religion, age, ethnicity, and profession. Gender is a facet of who we are—nothing more and nothing less. At this stage, the leader recognizes that attributing greater or lesser expertise to either sex, particularly with arrogance, is inadvertently to create yet another imbalance of power and barrier to service.

Burning with a clear blue flame is neither a static state nor a final destination. It is freedom to lead with clarity and purpose, perhaps in just brief moments at first, and then with ever-increasing frequency. In the words of South African President Nelson Mandela at his 1995 inaugural address: "As we are liberated from our own fear, our presence automatically liberates others."

Best wishes on your own journey to contribution, health, authenticity, and power—in service of others and yourself.

Appendix A: Contributors

· ·

Partial List of Contributors to
Women and Leadership in Health Care

Michael Annison
President
The Westrend Group Ltd.
Denver, Colorado

Eunice Azzani
Vice President and Partner
Korn/Ferry International
San Francisco, California

Geraldine Polly Bednash, PhD, RN, FAAN
Executive Director
American Association of Colleges of Nursing
Washington, D.C.

Hudson H. Birden, Jr., MPH
Director of Health
City of New Britain, Connecticut

Heidi Boerstler, JD, DrPH
Department Chair, Programs in Health Administration
University of Colorado
Denver, Colorado

Linda Burnes Bolton, RN, DRPH
Director, Nursing Resources
Cedars-Sinai Medical Center
Los Angeles, California

Robert and Carolyn Boyle
Consultants and Former Hospital and Group Practice Executives
Frisco, Texas

Pamela Bromley, MSN, RN
Vice President, Patient Care Services
Saint Alphonsus Regional Medical Center
Boise, Idaho

Connie Burgess, MSN, RN
Burgess and Associates
Lakewood, California

Lawton R. Burns, PhD
Associate Professor of Healthcare Systems
Wharton School, University of Pennsylvania
Philadelphia, Pennsylvania

Jeffrey B. Caballero, MPH
Associate Director, Internal Programs
Association of Asian Pacific Community Health Organizations
Oakland, California

Patricia A. Cahill, JD
President & Chief Executive Officer
Catholic Health Initiatives
Denver, Colorado

Leanne Kaiser Carlson, MSHA
Kaiser and Associates
Brighton, Colorado

Dolores G. Clement, DrPH
Associate Dean, School of Allied Health Professions
Virginia Commonwealth University/Medical College of Virginia
Richmond, Virginia

Elaine Cohen, EdD, RN
Director of Case Management/Associate Professor
University of Colorado Health Sciences Center
Denver, Colorado

Vince Covello, PhD
Covello Communications
New York, New York

Molly Joel Coye, MD, MPH
Director
The Lewin Group
San Francisco, California

Anne Hall Davis
Community Trustee
Harwich Port, Massachusetts

Robert A. DeVries
Program Director
W.K. Kellogg Foundation
Battlecreek, Michigan

Joy Dobson, RN, MS
Healthy Community Coordinator
Petaluma Health Care District
Petaluma, California

Barbara Donaho, RN, MA, FAAN
Health Consultant and Retired Healthcare Executive
St. Petersburg, Florida

Catherine Dower, JD
Health Law and Policy Analyst
Center for the Health Professions
University of California
San Francisco, California

Karen S. Ehrat, PhD, RN
Senior Vice President MRHS-GC
President, Mercy Hospitals, Anderson/Clermont
Cincinnati, Ohio

Henry Fernandez, JD
Former President
Association of University Programs in Health Administration
Washington, D.C.

Maura Fields, BSN, RN
Director, Professional Services
North Valley Hospital
White Fish, Montana

David J. Fine, MHA
Regents Professor and Chairman
School of Public Health and Tropical Medicine
Tulane University Medical Center
New Orleans, Louisiana

Leonard J. Finocchio, MPH
Associate Director
Center for the Health Professions
University of California
San Francisco, California

Donna Fosbinder, DNS, RN
Associate Professor, Coordinator
Graduate Program in Nursing Administration
Brigham Young University
Provo, Utah

Deborah A. Freund, PhD
Vice Chancellor for Academic Affairs
University of Indiana
Bloomington, Indiana

Alain Gauthier and Joan Kenley, PhD
Core Leadership Development Group
Oakland, California

Lillee Gelinias, RN, MSN
Vice President, Clinical Improvement Services
VHA, Inc.
Irving, Texas

Elaina Spitaels Genser
Partner, Witt/Kieffer, Ford, Hadelman, Lloyd
Emeryville, California

Jeff Goldsmith, PhD
Consultant and Author
Charlottesville, Pennsylvania

Adela Gonzalez, MPH
Associate Vice President, Multicultural Affairs
Assistant Director, Public Health Program
University of North Texas, Health Sciences Center
Austin, Texas

William Gonzalez
President & Chief Executive Officer
Butterworth Health System
Grand Rapids, Michigan

Fred E. Graham, PhD, CAE
President, AudioWorks
Former Associate Director, Medical Group Management
Association
Denver, Colorado

Cynthia Carter Haddock, PhD
Professor and Director, MSHA Program
Department of Health Service Administration
University of Alabama at Birmingham
Birmingham, Alabama

Joseph M. Hafey, MPH
President and CEO
Public Health Institute
Berkeley, California

Patrick G. Hays
President & CEO
Blue Cross/Blue Shield Association
Chicago, Illinois

Sandra Hernandez, MD
Chief Executive Officer
San Francisco Foundation
San Francisco, California

Bettsanne Homes
Immediate Past Chairwoman
Volunteer Trustees
Falmouth, Maine

Myra Isenhart, PhD
Principal, Organizational Communications, Inc.
Denver, Colorado

Kathryn E. Johnson
President & Chief Executive Officer
The Healthcare Forum
San Francisco, California

Doloras Jones, MS, RN
Senior Vice President
Kaiser Foundation Hospital
Former President, Organization of California Nurse Executives
Oakland, California

Wanda Jones, MPH
President, New Century Healthcare Institute
San Francisco, California

Leland R. Kaiser, PhD
President
Kaiser and Associates
Brighton, Colorado

Sumedna M. Khanna, MD, MPH
Executive Director, Healing Well Associates
Fremont, California

David A. Kindig, MD, PhD
President, Board of Directors
Association of Health Services Research
Chair, Council on Graduate Medical Education
Professor, Department of Preventative Medicine
School of Medicine, University of Wisconsin
Madison, Wisconsin

Alma L. Koch, PhD, MPH
Associate Director
Graduate School of Public Health
San Diego State University
San Diego, California

JoEllen Koerner, RN, MA, FAAN, PhD
Former Chair, American Organization of Nurse Executives
Former Vice President of Patient Services
Sioux Valley Hospital
Sioux Valley, South Dakota

Jennifer L. Kozakowski, MPH
Associate Director of Client Services
Value Health Sciences, Inc.
Los Angeles, California

Phyllis Kritek, PhD, RN
Author and Professor, School of Nursing, Medical Branch
University of Texas
Galveston, Texas

Nancy M. Lakier, MBA, RN
Partner
Innovia Health
San Diego, California

Lynne Langdon
Vice President, Sub-Specialty Department
Director of Examination Development
American Board of Internal Medicine
Philadelphia, Pennsylvania

Sharon Lee, RN, BSBA, CNAA, FACHE
Senior Vice President, Patient Care Services
St. Luke's Regional Medical Center
Boise, Idaho

Diane Littlefield, MPH
Director, Center for Collaborative Planning
Sacramento, California

Cynthia Madden, PhD
Professor, Graduate Program
School of Public Health and Community Medicine
University of Washington
Seattle, Washington

Stephanie S. McCutcheon, MHA
Regional President and System Vice President
SSM Health Care System
St. Louis, Missouri

Gates McKibbin, PhD
Consultant
San Francisco, California

Cathleen Michaels, RN, PhD, FAAN
Post-Doctoral Fellow, Community-Based Interventions
College of Nursing, University of Arizona
Tucson, Arizona

Judith R. Miller, RN
Senior Fellow, Institute for Healthcare Improvement
Former Chair, American Organization of Nurse Executives
Boston, Massachusetts

Linda Miller
President
Volunteer Trustees
Washington, DC

Margaret Neale, PhD
Professor, Graduate School of Business
Stanford University
Stanford, California

Jane Neubauer, MN, RN
Fellow, King's Fund College of London
President, The Creative Leadership Retreat
Vashon Island, Washington

Carmen Rita Nevarez, MD
Vice President for External Relations
Public Health Institute
Berkeley, California

Gregory Oliva, MPH
Outreach Coordinator
Cardiovascular Disease Outreach Resource
and Epidemiology Program
California Department of Health Services
Sacramento, California

Edward M. O'Neil, PhD
Executive Director
Center for Health Professions
University of California
San Francisco, California

Mary Pittman, DrPH
President, Hospital Research and Educational Trust
Chicago, Illinois

Dennis D. Pointer, PhD
Hanlon Professor of Health Services Management
San Diego State University
San Diego, California

Peter A. Rabinowitz
President, PAR Associates, Inc.
Boston, Massachusetts

Kathy Reno, RN, MBA
Vice President, Clinical Services
Northwest Community Healthcare
Chicago, Illinois

Mary Richardson, PhD
Director, Graduate Program in Health
Services Administration and Planning
School of Public Health and Community Medicine
University of Washington
Seattle, Washington

Walt Rosebrough
President and Chief Executive Officer
Hill-Rom Corporation
Batesville, Indiana

Sr. Mary Jean Ryan
President & Chief Executive Officer
SSM Health System
St. Louis, Missouri

Doug Scutchfield, MD
Director, Division of Health Services Management
University of Kentucky
Louisville, Kentucky

Joel Shalowitz, MD, MM, FACP
Professor and Program Director, Health Services Management
Kellogg Graduate School of Management
Northwestern University
Chicago, Illinois

Stephen Shortell, PhD
Blue Cross Distinguished Professor
of Health Policy and Management
Professor of Organizational Behavior
School of Public Health, University of California
Berkeley, California

Carol Spain, MPH
Director, Public Health Leadership Institute
Centers for Disease Control and
Prevention/University of California
Berkeley, California

Roxane Spitzer, PhD, MBA, RN, FAAN
Professor and Associate Dean for Practice Management
School of Nursing
Vanderbilt University
Knoxville, Tennessee

Eileen Sporing, MSN, RN
Vice President, Patient Services
Children's Hospital
Boston, Massachusetts

Dennis W. Strum, PhD
President, The Strum Group
Los Angeles, California

Jane W. Swanson, MS, RN, CNAA
Retired Captain, Navy Nurse Corps
Former Associate Director, Nursing
National Naval Medical Center
Bethesda, Maryland

Pamela Austin Thompson, RN, MSN
Vice President, Dartmouth-Hitchcock Medical Center
President of the Board, New Hampshire Hospital Association
Lebanon, New Hampshire

Nancy Valentine, PhD, RN, MPH, FAAN
Chief Consultant, Nursing Strategic Health Care Group
Department of Veterans Affairs
Washington, DC

Victoria Breckwith Vasquez, MPH
Health Educator/Training Specialist
University Health Service
University of California
Berkeley, California

Katherine W. Vestal, PhD, RN, FAAN
National Director, Work Transformation Services
Hay Management Consultants
Dallas, Texas

The late Duane D. Walker, RN, MS, FAAN
Former Vice President, Patient Services
The Queen's Medical Center
Honolulu, Hawaii

Myrna Warnick, PhD, RN
Professor, Graduate Program in Nursing Administration
Brigham Young University
Provo, Utah

Carla Wiggins, PhD
Assistant Dean, Program Chairperson
Health and Human Management
Franklin University
Columbus, Ohio

Anne Witmer, MPH
Former Program Coordinator
Centers for Disease Control and Prevention/University of
California Public Health Leadership Institute
Berkeley, California

Donna Wright, RN, MS
Staff Development Specialist/Consultant
Creative Healthcare Management
Minneapolis, Minnesota

Nando Zepeda, MAEd., MBA, MPH
Retired Manager, Organizational Development
Los Angeles County Department of Health Services
Los Angeles, California

Appendix B: Demographics

1997 Gender and Leadership in Healthcare Study: Demographic Characteristics of Study Participants

Number of contributors (answering some or all study questions)	82	
Males	22	(27 percent)
Females	60	(73 percent)
Degrees obtained		
MD	5	(6 percent)
RN	31	(37 percent)
MS (not terminal degree)	36	(44 percent)
MS (terminal degree)	20	(24 percent)
PhD	34	(41 percent)
PhD (with another doctoral degree or equivalent)	2	(2 percent)
JD	3	(4 percent)
BA	1	(1 percent)
Minorities	7	(9 percent)
Male	2	
Female	5	
African American	1	
Hispanic	5	
Indian	1	

Age ranges at time of study:

31–35	2	(2 percent)
36–40	3	(4 percent)
41–45	17	(21 percent)
46–50	24	(29 percent)
51–55	23	(28 percent)
56–60	8	(10 percent)
60+	5	(6 percent)

Appendix C: Data

. . . .

1997 Gender and Leadership in Healthcare Study: Key Questions and Numerical Results

Do you think gender plays a major role in leadership practice in health care? If so, please elaborate.

Total respondents = 75 (91 percent of sample total of 82 study contributors who were asked this question)

Yes	69	(92 percent)
No	4	(5 percent)
Don't know	2	(3 percent)
Males	20	(27 percent)
Yes	18	(90 percent)
No	1	(5 percent)
Don't know	1	(5 percent)
Females	55	(73 percent)
Yes	51	(91 percent)
No	2	(4 percent)
Don't know	2	(4 percent)

Note: These data reflect only yes/no answers. All study questions were optional and open-ended, so contributors supplied interpretations as well as these responses.

*Do you notice differences in effective leadership behaviors between
male and female clinical leaders and other healthcare executives?
(Your answer should be based on your own definition of effective.)
If so, what are they?*

Total respondents = 69 (84 percent of sample total)

Yes		52 (75 percent)
No		17 (25 percent)
Not included		1
Males		19 (27 percent)
	Yes	9 (47 percent)
	No	10 (53 percent)
Females		49 (73 percent)
	Yes	41 (84 percent)
	No	8 (16 percent)

*Do you think gender plays a major role in your own leadership
practice? As you have evolved as a leader, has that role changed?*

Total respondents = 52 (63 percent of sample total)

Yes		43 (83 percent)
No		9 (17 percent)
Males		9 (17 percent)
	Yes	5 (56 percent)
	No	4 (44 percent)
Females		43 (83 percent)
	Yes	38 (88 percent)
	No	5 (12 percent)

*Do you think gender makes more or less difference now, in these times
of so much change in healthcare? Please say more.*

Total respondents = 46 (56 percent of sample total)

More		12 (26 percent)
Less		19 (41 percent)
Same		9 (20 percent)
Other		6 (13 percent)
Males		13 (28 percent)
	More	4 (31 percent)
	Less	8 (62 percent)
	Same	1 (8 percent)
	Other	1 (8 percent)
Females		33 (72 percent)
	More	8 (24 percent)
	Less	11 (33 percent)
	Same	8 (24 percent)
	Other	6 (18 percent)

References

• •

Aburdene, P., and Naisbitt, J. *Megatrends for Women: From Liberation to Leadership*. New York: Fawcett Columbine, 1992.

American College of Healthcare Executives (ACHE) and Graduate Program in Hospital and Health Administration. *Gender and Careers in Healthcare Management: Findings of a National Survey of Healthcare Executives*. Chicago, Illinois, 1991.

American College of Healthcare Executives and Graduate Program in Hospital and Health Administration. *A Comparison of the Career Attainments of Men and Women Healthcare Executives*. Chicago, Illinois, 1996.

Argyris, C. "Teaching Smart People How to Learn." *Harvard Business Review*, May-June 1991, pp. 99–109.

Bennis, W. "Leadership Theory and Administrative Behavior." *Administrative Science Quarterly*, 1996, *4*, 259–260.

Bennis, W. Presentation. University Southern California Leadership Symposium. San Francisco, California, Apr. 1996.

Borysenko, J. *A Woman's Book of Life: The Biology, Psychology, and Spirituality of the Feminine Life Cycle*. New York: Riverhead Books, 1996.

Bridges, W. *Transitions: Making Sense of Life's Changes*. Reading, Mass.: Addison-Wesley, 1980.

Bridges, W. *Jobshift: How to Prosper in a Workplace Without Jobs*. Reading, Mass.: Addison-Wesley, 1995.

Briles, J. *Gender Traps*. New York: McGraw-Hill, 1996.

Brown, J., Isaacs, D., and others. *The Systems Thinker*, Dec. 1996, 7(10).

Campbell, J. *The Wisdom of Joseph Campbell: A Retrospective* (1975–1987). Audio Tape Series, New Dimensions, 1997.

Capozzalo, G., Bisognano, E., Gaucher, E., Ryan, M. J., Sr. "The Glass Ceiling in Health Care: A Round Table Discussion." *Quality Connection*, Fall 1995, 4(4), 1–3.

Collins, J. C., and Porras, J. *Built to Last: Successful Habits of Visionary Companies*. New York: HarperBusiness, 1994.

Cooper, R. K., and Sawaf, A. *Executive EQ: Emotional Intelligence in Leadership and Organizations*. New York: Grosset/Putnam, 1997.

Csikszentmihalyi, M. *Flow*. New York: Harper & Row, 1990.

Dreachslin, J. L. *Diversity Leadership*. Chicago: Health Administration Press, 1996.

Dreher, G. F., and Ash, R. A. "A Comparative Study of Mentoring Among Men and Women in Managerial, Professional and Technical Positions." *Journal of Applied Psychology*, Oct. 1990, 75(5), 539–546.

Duff, C. S. *When Women Work Together: Using Our Strengths to Overcome Our Challenges*. Berkeley, Calif.: Conari Press, 1993.

Eisler, R. *The Chalice and the Blade: Our History, Our Future*. San Francisco: Harper & Row, 1987.

Eubanks, P. "Key Players Must Help Shatter the Glass Ceiling, Say Experts. *Hospitals*, 65(19), Oct. 5, 1991, pp. 17–21.

Feudenberger, H. *Burnout: How to Beat the High Cost of Success*. New York: Doubleday, 1980.

Franklin, D. "What Your Voice Says About You." *Health*, Jan.–Feb. 1995, pp. 38–41.

Frantz, R., and Pattakos, A. N. *Intuition at Work: Pathways to Unlimited Possibilities*. San Francisco: Sterling and Stone, 1996.

Friedman, E. (ed.). *An Unfinished Revolution: Women and Health Care in America*. New York: United Hospital Fund of New York, 1994.

Gardner, J. "Self Renewal." *The Futurist*. Nov.–Dec. 1996, p. 10.

Gibson, R. (ed.). *Rethinking the Future: Rethinking Business, Principles, Competition, Control and Complexity, Leadership, Markets, and the World*. London: Nicholas Brealey Publishing, 1997.

Gilligan, C. *In a Different Voice: Psychological Theory and Women's Development*. Cambridge, Mass.: Harvard University Press, 1982.

Goss, T. *The Last Word on Power: Executive Re-invention for Leaders Who Must Make the Impossible Happen*. New York: Doubleday Currency, 1996.

Gruenfeld, D. H., Mannix, E. A., Williams, K. Y., and Neale, M. A. "Group Composition and Decision Making: How Member Familiarity and Information Distribution Affect Process and Performance." *Organizational Behavior and Human Decision Process*, July 1996, 67(1), 1–15.

Huang, C. A., and Lynch, J. *Mentoring: The Tao of Giving and Receiving Wisdom*. San Francisco: HarperSanFrancisco, 1995.

Isaacs, W. "Dialogue: The Power of Collective Thinking." *The Systems Thinker*, Apr. 1997, 3(4), 1–4.

Isenhart, M. "Mentoring for a Change: From Homer to Healthcare." *Medical Group Management Journal*, Sept.–Oct. 1996, 43(5), 78, 80–90.

Jaworski, J. *Synchronicity: The Inner Path of Leadership*. San Francisco: Berrett-Koehler, 1996.

Jones, W. J. *"The Healthcare Delivery System of the Future: Ignore, Watch or Create?"* San Francisco: New Century Healthcare Institute, 1997.

Kanter, R. M. *Men and Women of the Corporation*. New York: Basic Books, 1977.

Kao, J. *Jamming: The Art and Discipline of Corporate Creativity*. New York: HarperBusiness, 1997.

Kenley, J. *Voice Power*. New York: Henry Holt, 1988.

Klenke, K. *Women and Leadership: A Contextual Perspective*. New York: Springer, 1996.

Koerner, J. "The Reflective Executive: An Inner Journey of Inquiry." Presentation to the Center for Nursing Leadership, Batesville, Ind., Oct. 1996.

Korn/Ferry International. *Developing Leadership for the 21st Century*. 1996.

Kritek, P. B. *Negotiating at an Uneven Table: Developing Moral Courage in Resolving Our Conflicts*. San Francisco: Jossey-Bass, 1994.

Laing, M. "Gossip: Does It Play a Role in the Socialization of Nurses?" *Image: The Journal of Nursing Scholarship*, 1993, *1*(25), pp. 37–43.

Lipman-Blumen, J. *The Connective Edge: Leading in an Interdependent World*. San Francisco: Jossey-Bass, 1996.

Marcus, L. J., and others. *Renegotiating Health Care: Resolving Conflict to Build Collaboration*. San Francisco: Jossey-Bass, 1995.

Miller, J. B. *Toward a New Psychology of Women*. (2nd ed.). Boston: Beacon Press, 1997.

Murphy, E. C. *Leadership IQ*. New York: Wiley, 1996.

Neuhauser, P. *Tribal Warfare in Organizations: Turning Tribal Conflict into Negotiated Peace*. New York: HarperBusiness, 1988.

Neuhauser, P. *Corporate Legends and Lore: The Power of Storytelling as a Management Tool*. New York: McGraw-Hill, 1993.

Noer, D. M. *Breaking Free: A Prescription for Personal and Organizational Change*. San Francisco: Jossey-Bass, 1996.

Parker, V. A., and Kram, K. E. "Women Mentoring Women: Creating Conditions for Connection." *Business Horizons*, Mar.–Apr. 1993, 36(2), 42–51.

Paul, M. *The Systems Thinker*, Feb. 1997, 8(1), p. 1.

Pearson, C. S. *The Hero Within: Six Archetypes We Live By*. San Francisco: HarperSanFrancisco, 1989.

Rivers, F. *The Way of the Owl: Succeeding with Integrity in a Conflicted World*. San Francisco: HarperSanFrancisco, 1996.

Roberts, S. J. "Oppressed Group Behavior: Implications for Nursing." *Advances in Nursing Science*, July 1983, pp. 21–30.

Robinson, C. A. "Communication, Information and Leadership in a New Era." Curriculum module for the Public Health Leadership Institute, 1993–1996.

Rosener, J. B. "Ways Women Lead." *Harvard Business Review*, Nov.–Dec. 1990, pp. 119–125.

Rosener, J. B. *America's Competitive Secret: Utilizing Women as a Management Strategy*. New York: Oxford University Press, 1995.

Ryan, S. Presentation to the Center for Nursing Leadership. Pleasanton, Calif., Oct. 15, 1996.

Sheehy, G. *New Passages: Mapping Your Life Across Time*. New York: Random House, 1995.

Sinetar, M. *The Mentor Spirit*. Tape Series. Sounds True. Boulder, Colorado, 1997.

Spitzer, R. *Gender Influences and Issues in the Workplace*. Emergency Department Management Manual: Principles and Application, 1997, pp. 729–733.

Tannen, D. *You Just Don't Understand: Women and Men in Conversation*. New York: Morrow, 1990.

Tannen, D. *Talking from 9 to 5*. New York: Morrow, 1994.

Tavris, C. *The Mismeasure of Women: Why Women Are Not the Better Sex, the Inferior Sex or the Opposite Sex*. New York: Touchstone Books, 1993.

Taylor, D. *The Healing Power of Stories: Creating Yourself Through the Stories of Your Life*. New York: Doubleday, 1996.

Thin Elk, G. Presentation to the Center for Nursing Leadership. Pleasanton, Calif., Oct. 1996.

Weil, P., and others. "Exploring the Gender Gap in Healthcare Management." *Healthcare Executive*, Nov.–Dec. 1996.

Webber, A.M. "What's So New About the New Economy?" *Harvard Business Review*, Jan.–Feb. 1993, p. 24.

Wilbur, K. *A Brief History of Everything*. Boston: Shambhala, 1996.

Index